The Patient's Guide To Heart Valve Surgery

By

Adam Pick

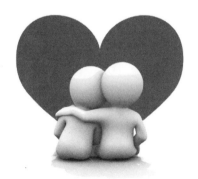

The Patient's Guide To Heart Valve Surgery

Avoid stress. Know what to expect. Enhance recovery.

by

Adam Pick
Double Heart Valve Surgery Patient

Revised Edition

The Patient's Guide To Heart Valve Surgery

P.O. Box 1671
El Segundo, CA 90245
adam@Heart-Valve-Surgery.com
http://www.Heart-Valve-Surgery.com

LIMIT OF LIABILITY/DISCLAIMER OF WARRANTY:

Author and publisher have used their best efforts in preparing this book. The author and publisher make no representations or warranties with respect to the accuracy or completeness of the contents of this book and specifically disclaim any implied warranties of merchantability or fitness for a particular purpose. There are no warranties that extend beyond the descriptions contained in this paragraph. No warranty may be created or extended by sales representatives or written sales materials.

The accuracy and completeness of the information provided herein and the opinions stated herein are not guaranteed or warranted to produce any particular results, and the advice and strategies contained herein may not be suitable for every individual. Neither author nor publisher shall be liable for any loss of profit or any other commercial damages, including but not limited to special, incidental, consequential, or other damages.

The content in this book is not intended as a substitute for medical or professional counseling advice. The reader is encouraged to continually consult his or her physician on all health matters, especially symptoms that may require professional diagnosis and/or medical attention.

TRADEMARKS

All brand names and product names used in this book and web site are trade names, service marks, trademarks, or registered trademarks of their respective owners.

THE INTERNET

To the best of our knowledge, all web site unified resource locators (URLs) listed in this web site are correct at the time of publishing. With the Internet changing daily, please excuse any URL errors due to these changes.

Library of Congress Cataloging-in-Publication Data
Pick, Adam
The Patient's Guide To Heart Valve Surgery: Know what to expect. Avoid stress. Enhance recovery.
Library of Congress Control Number: 2007904222
1. Patient self-help 2. Heart valve surgery 3. Surgery recovery

Book layout designed by Lynne Talbot, www.lynnetalbot.com

ISBN 978-0-615-14703-1

Printed in United States of America

Patient, Caregiver and Doctor Testimonials

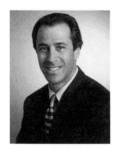

I strongly encourage patients and caregivers to read *The Patient's Guide To Heart Valve Surgery*. This book offers unique and knowledgeable insight into heart valve surgery from the patient's perspective. There is much to gain from Adam Pick's research.

— Doctor, Marc Darrow, MD, California
Board Certified Physiatrist Specializing in Rehabilitation

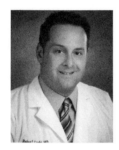

A patient's realistic understanding of their pending medical procedure enables them to obtain a sense of control over their expectations which ultimately results in an efficient and healthy recovery. For that reason, *The Patient's Guide To Heart Valve Surgery* is an effective resource for cardiac surgery patients.

— Doctor, Robert T. Light, MD, Virginia
Diplomat of the American Board of Psychiatry and Neurology

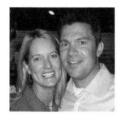

Your book is the reason my surgery went so well. Thank you so much! I think every patient facing valve surgery should read *The Patient's Guide To Heart Valve Surgery*.

— Patient, Taylor Browning, California

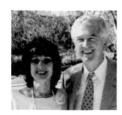

This is a wonderful book. The integration of clinical information and personal experience provides the reader with a holistic picture of the realities of heart valve surgery.

— Caregiver, Donna Pearson, California

More Patient and Caregiver Testimonials...

I read *The Patient's Guide To Heart Valve Surgery* the day I bought it. The book was very informative as I am currently evaluating the best valve surgery for me. The book also shed some different light on what to expect during the recovery from heart valve surgery.

— Patient, Roger Sudbeck, South Dakota

Thank you for sharing your candid thoughts and experiences! I require an aortic valve replacement and your book has been a great source of information. Thank you and stay healthy.

— Patient, John Vardy, Al Khor, Qatar

The Patient's Guide To Heart Valve Surgery was enlightening. There was a great deal of information in it that you would not get from the medical profession.

— Patient, Robert Waterman, Connecticut

I just want to thank you. My uncle received *The Patient's Guide To Heart Valve Surgery* on Saturday and was very impressed. I only wish he had your book BEFORE his surgery. He really appreciated your patient perspective on heart valve surgery.

— Caregiver, Diane Kendrick, Eugene, Oregon

I am very impressed with *The Patient's Guide To Heart Valve Surgery*. It gave me a good view of what to expect and to watch out for. I am sure it will be a big benefit to my experience and recovery. Thanks for sharing your experience and knowledge with others.

— Patient, John Riordan, Centerport, New York

Both Colleen (my wife) and I have read *The Patient's Guide To Heart Valve Surgery*. Speaking of the drug issue, I believe you make some good points in the book about the necessity of dealing with pain management issues without getting too dependent on pain killers.

— Patient, Philip Bonds, Kremmling, Colorado

What Do Heart Surgeons Think About
The Patient's Guide To Heart Valve Surgery?

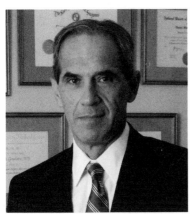

**Dr. Vincent Gaudiani, M.D.,
Senior Cardiac Surgeon, Pacific Coast
Cardiac & Vascular Surgeons.**

Over the past 25 years,
Dr. Gaudiani has performed
over 10,000 procedures.

"Very impressive...
This book educates and supports patients."
—Dr. Luca Vricella, M.D.,
Cardiothoracic Surgeon,
The Johns Hopkins Hospital

"This book will help many patients – from
diagnosis through recovery."
—Dr. Gosta Pettersson, M.D., Ph.D.
Vice Chairman Of The Cleveland Clinic's Department
Of Thoracic And Cardiovascular Surgery

"Adam: Many patients are benefiting
from your work."
—Dr. Vincent Gaudiani, M.D., Senior Cardiac Surgeon,
Pacific Coast Cardiac & Vascular Surgeons

"I am very impressed by what you have created.
I would love to have your ideas incorporated into the
big conversation we seek to stimulate on my show."
— Dr. Mehmet Oz, M.D., Professor of Surgery,
New York-Presbyterian Hospital,
Host of "The Dr. Oz Show"

"I will find your book useful in explaining surgery.
It is most helpful."
—Dr. Donald Ross, M.D.,
Inventor of The Ross Procedure

"Quite remarkable... I appreciate this book."
—Dr. Kevin Accola, M.D., Cardiac Surgeon,
Cardiovascular Surgeons, P.A. (Florida)

Do You Recognize The Names Of These Former Heart Valve Surgery Patients?

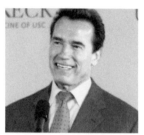

Arnold Schwarzenegger celebrated his ten-year anniversary of heart valve surgery on April 16, 2007 at the Keck School of Medicine at USC.
(Photo: Jon Nalick)

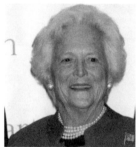

On March 4, 2009, Barbara Bush, Former First Lady of the United States, had aortic valve surgery. (Source: PR Photo)

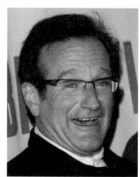

On March 13, 2009, Robin Williams had aortic and mitral valve surgery.
(Source: PR Photo)

Arnold Schwarzenegger
(Actor/Governor)

Robin Williams
(Actor/Comedian)

Barbara Bush
(Former First Lady
of The United States)

Elizabeth Taylor
(Actress)

Ed Koch
(Former New York City Mayor)

Jim Lehrer
(Television News Anchor)

Charlie Rose
(Journalist)

Jesse Helms
(Senator)

Rodney Dangerfield
(Comedian)

Teppo Numminen
(Professional Hockey Star)

Aaron Boone
(Professional Baseball Star)

Adam Pick, author of
The Patient's Guide To Heart Valve Surgery,
comments on the purpose of this unique book:

"In a recent survey of 78 former heart valve surgery patients, most respondents suggested that recovering from heart valve surgery was *more difficult than expected...*

"In that same survey, more than **41% of patients felt their cardiologist and surgeon could have better prepared them for heart valve surgery recovery.**

"My own patient experience compelled me to learn more and to help future patients and caregivers. *This book was designed with three key objectives - to help patients manage their expectations, to help patients minimize their stress and to help patients accelerate their recovery.*"

About the Author – Adam Pick

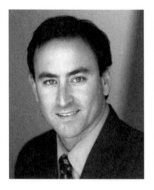

As one of the leading analysts in his field, Adam Pick has been featured in *The Wall Street Journal, BusinessWeek, CIO Magazine, The Economist* and several other publications for his unique knowledge of electronics manufacturing.

A native of Los Angeles, Adam earned a Bachelor of Arts and a Masters of Business Administration from the University of Michigan.

On November 3, 2005, Adam was diagnosed with severe heart valve disease. Eight weeks later, Dr. Vaughn Starnes performed aortic and pulmonary valve replacements (via the *Ross Procedure*) on Mr. Pick at the University of Southern California Medical Center.

After a long and difficult recovery, Adam is back to work, exercising five times per week and traveling the world for fun and business. Adam's heart valve surgery success story was elevated on July 7, 2007 when he married Robyn Podell, his girlfriend of two years. In 2009, Adam and Robyn celebrated the birth of their first child, Ethan.

As part of his experience with heart valve surgery, Adam learned the highs, the lows, the challenges, the opportunities and the frustrations of heart valve surgery. This book is his attempt to guide and support patients and caregivers through the entire heart valve surgery process — from diagnosis to recovery.

Adam Pick provides on-going comments specific to heart valve surgery and recovery at his personal blog located at http://www.heart-valve-surgery.com/heart-surgery-blog/.

Dedication

This book is dedicated to every human, every doctor, every nurse, every researcher, every pharmaceutical company, every medical device manufacturer and every patient that has furthered the pursuit of healthy hearts.

This book is also dedicated to my friends and family who visited me in room 550 at USC Medical Center, who sat in traffic on the 405 Freeway in Los Angeles and who crossed the country by plane to be with me and support me. You — Donna, Al, Jerry, Judie, Sylvia, Doug, Susie, Ellie, Monica, Robert, Buddy, Mimi, Marc, Michelle, Rob, Rachel, Bonnie, and John Roger — are the source of my restored ability to smile and laugh.

To Dr. Starnes, you truly are the *Michael Jordan* of heart valve surgery.

To Dr. Rosin, thanks for listening to me and my heart. You are an amazing cardiologist.

Cheers to Debbie, Karey, Donna, Socorro, Sidney and Sherri at Torrance Memorial's Cardiac Rehab Program. Collectively, you strengthened my body and recharged my mind.

Thanks to each of the seventy-eight, former heart valve surgery patients and caregivers that participated in my online survey about heart valve surgery. Your stories touched, moved and inspired me.

A special thanks to my management team and co-workers at iSuppli. Your support and understanding during my recovery was extraordinary.

Lastly to Robyn, there are no boundaries for the love and indebtedness I have for you. You are simply amazing.

New Free Online Tools for Patients & Caregivers...

Designed Exclusively For The Heart Valve Surgery Community!

The Heart Valve Surgeon Database. Finding a trusted, heart valve surgeon can be a very difficult and time-consuming process. For this reason, the patient and caregiver community at www.Heart-Valve-Surgery.com decided to create a FREE heart surgeon database. This special directory contains (i) global surgeon listings and (ii) actual patient experiences with heart valve surgeons. Ultimately, the database was developed to help you find reputable heart valve surgeons quickly!

To get direct patient feedback about heart valve surgeons from around the world, please go to **www.HeartValveSurgeons.com.**

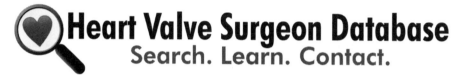

Heart Valve Journals. To help patients stay connected with their caregivers throughout the entire heart valve surgery experience, Adam Pick recently launched a free, online tool known as Heart Valve Journals.

Now, with Heart Valve Journals, patients can keep their support group updated at all times. From diagnosis through recovery, patients can write journals, post pictures and share stories. Plus, caregivers can interact with patients through a special Internet feature known as the *Guestbook*.

Finally, Heart Valve Journals provide a unique opportunity for patients to meet and learn from other patients all over the world.

To create your free journal, please go to **www.HeartValveJournals.com.**

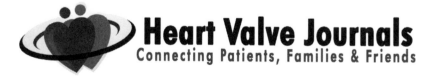

Table of Contents

PART 1 – LEARNING ABOUT HEART VALVE SURGERY

PART 2 – PREPARING FOR HEART VALVE SURGERY

PART 3 – THE HEART VALVE OPERATION

PART I

LEARNING ABOUT HEART VALVE SURGERY

Dispelling The Fear Of Heart Surgery!

In this chapter, you will:
- Learn how to manage your fear relating to heart valve surgery.
- Understand the facts about heart valve surgery.
- Feel better about the next steps of this experience.

As a heart valve surgery patient, I can imagine what you may be going through right now. I can imagine that you may be confused. I can imagine that you may be nervous. And, I can imagine that you are experiencing a unique type of fear that you have never felt before. Lastly, I can also imagine that several questions are racing through your mind. The questions I remember were:

- Why me?
- Do I *really* need to have heart valve surgery?
- Will I ever be the same again?
- How painful will the operation be?
- And the big question...Will I die?

While I could continue this list of questions, I am not going to.

Don't worry. There will be a time and place to ask those questions. But, this is not that time. And, this is not the place.

Instead, I want to spend the opening of this book on a warm, positive note. I want to give you some medical assurances. I want to let you know that you are in good hands. And, I want to let you know that if I can survive a *double heart valve replacement* procedure, so can you!

"How is Adam going to dispel my fears about open heart surgery?" you may be thinking.

Well, let me start by providing you with well-documented facts about heart valve surgery.

 Facts #1 and #2 – Each year, over 700,000 heart surgeries take place across the world. Of those surgeries, more than 250,000 are valve surgeries.

What do these facts tell you? First, they tell you that you are not alone. There are many people out there just like you. So, try not to feel that heart valve surgery is your challenge only. Support groups and recovery centers are waiting to help you before, during and after the surgery.

Second, I share these facts because it should make you feel better about the medical procedure that awaits you. Whichever procedure you choose, please know you are not the first person to 'test' it out. The odds are pretty high that your entire medical staff has already performed this operation not once, but hundreds of times.

 Fact #3 – The mortality rate for heart valve surgery is only 2.4%.

That's right. I did just provide you with the *real big fact* about heart valve surgery. Now, it's your turn to process that fact.

But, wait!!!

Before you do that, consider that the mortality rate has dropped significantly during the past twenty years. At some clinics, including The Cleveland Clinic, the mortality rate is only 2.4%.

Wait some more!!!

There's more good news to share.

You should also know that some minimally invasive heart surgery procedures have mortality rates that are close to zero percent.

Quick question: Are you feeling any better about heart valve surgery now?

It is true and unfortunate that some patients do not make it through the surgery. But, when you think about it, life is risk. From the moment you wake up in the morning, you are in a risky situation. Just consider the act of driving. I don't know about you, but I live in Los Angeles. The drivers here are crazy! At least once a week I yell out to someone, "What are you trying to kill me?"

 Fact #4 – Medical technology is on your side!

The world of medicine is changing everyday. One of the key reasons for that change is the advance of medical technology.

As you have just read, new procedures are being developed to enhance the patient's surgical experience. To give you an idea as to how quickly medical technology can impact heart valve operations, consider the recent acceptance of *minimally invasive valve replacement and repair surgery.*

Thanks to non-traditional surgical approaches (e.g. mini-sternotomy, thoracotomy) and robotic machines, heart valve surgery can be performed with an incision no longer than three inches. So you know, I have a nine-inch scar running down my sternum. That's a six-inch difference!

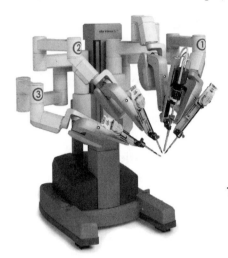

The da Vinci Surgical Robot For
Mitral Valve Repair
(Source: Intuitive Surgical)

Furthermore, there are new catheter-based approaches for heart valve repair and replacement surgery that require no sternum incision. Yes, you read that correct... No sternum incision!

Examples of these catheter-based technologies include the Edwards SAPIEN Valve for aortic and pulmonary valve replacement and the MitraClip for mitral valve repair. Both of these transcatheter solutions are already available for use in Europe. It is expected that the Food and Drug Administration (FDA) could approve these minimally invasive solutions in the United States within the next few years.

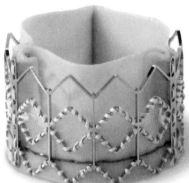

Edwards SAPIEN Valve
(Source: Edwards Lifesciences)

While these technologies have shown encouraging results, it is critical that patients fully understand that these procedures are *new* or *relatively new*. That said, surgical statistics – including success and failure rates - are still in development.

Dr. Vincent Gaudiani, a cardiac surgeon who has practiced for the past twenty-five years, addresses this point in his online video series, *How Should Patients Think About Surgical Outcomes?* (http://www.heart-valve-surgery.com/heart-surgery-blog/2009/09/10/video-dr-gaudiani-surgical-outcomes-mitral-valve/).

"We tend to be a society that is very impressed by new technology," notes Dr. Gaudiani, "But, not all new technology is effective – particularly in medical situations... Although new technology is very important, the older technology continues to improve."

Regardless of which procedure you and your surgeon agree upon, you are about to experience a medical miracle. Thanks to the technology - drugs, medical devices and robots - your experience will be much more comfortable than it would have been ten, or even five, years ago.

The Transformation Of Fear...

I am hopeful that you are starting to feel better about the reality of heart valve surgery in your life. While it is a very serious operation, the statistics suggest that you are going to be fine.

I know that might be a little hard to accept right now but, as you read this book and learn more about your procedure, your doctor, and your recovery, I believe you will start to see the benefits of this operation not the fear.

Your *'fear transformation'* may take months to occur.

Guess what? That's completely okay!

Just so you know... Before my operation, I interviewed a heart valve replacement patient who waited twelve months to have the operation. Eric was scared out of his mind – suffering from panic attacks and terrible anxiety.

Then, one year after his diagnosis, Eric changed his perception of the surgery.

Eight weeks later, Eric was back at work with a new, aortic heart valve.

Former Valve Surgery Patient Quote:
Sue Monks (United Kingdom)

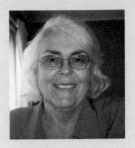

"Don't be frightened. If you die during the surgery you are not going to know anything about it. And, if you don't have the surgery you are going to die anyways. So, there is no point worrying about it!"

2

My Story – The Diagnosis

In this chapter, you will:
- · Relate to the emotions and experience of someone needing heart valve surgery.
- · Learn the details of my diagnosis.
- · Get inspired reading our *first* heart valve surgery success story.

I will never forget that first-and-only meeting with my new cardiologist, Dr. Bad Bedside Manner on November 3, 2005. He took a ten-second look at my echocardiogram results and said smugly, "Huh? Why weren't you here last year? Or, two years ago for that matter? You need a new valve! And, you need it soon."

The doctor continued to tell me that my heart was already *dilated* and suffering from 'working overtime' as he phrased it.

As I remember it now, time stood still in that white room with the white floors and that medical office smell. The walls were covered with heart posters, heart diagrams and other pharmaceutical-sponsored paraphernalia that related to my troubled heart.

I was numb. I was completely numb.

Dr. Bad Bedside Manner then took a fake, plastic heart that opened outward like a book and said, "Your aortic valve is really worn down." He continued with more medical, mumbo-jumbo that I did not understand.

This stoic man, with the red nose and short gray hair, did not make it any easier with his next comment. The doctor then said to me, "You're not going to die tomorrow but I would not wait more than six months to take care of this."

He then asked, "Have you fainted lately or gone numb on any part of your body recently?"

I instantly remembered that Mexican dinner with Robyn, my wife, a few weeks earlier. We had finished the first bowl of chips and salsa when the left side of my body went numb, very numb. A few seconds later, we were outside of the restaurant, walking to the car, destined for the hospital, when the numbness stopped.

"You are going to the doctor tomorrow!" Robyn pleaded with me.

Robyn knows I do not enjoy taking orders. So, she conveniently changed her command to a question, "Will you promise me that you will call for an appointment tomorrow?"

I acknowledged by nodding my head up and down.

I knew at that moment, it was time that I would have to undergo heart valve surgery. After years and years of waiting it was now time.

My Congenital Heart Murmur

Like many people, I was born with a *congenital heart defect*. When I was five years old, I was diagnosed with a bicuspid aortic valve. To make it easy on me, my parents told me that I had a *tiny heart murmur*. My mom and dad then comforted me by telling me that I was no different from the other children.

I really thought nothing of the heart murmur for the first twenty-six years of my life.

Every year, however, I would see a cardiologist for an annual echocardiogram. And, every year, my cardiologist would say, "Hmmm. The results are fine. Thanks for coming in. See you next year!"

Again, I thought nothing of my heart problem. All I knew was that I had a heart murmur and that my heartbeat was a little muffled.

In 1996, however, my cardiologist at the time, Dr. Richard Davison of Chicago's Northwestern Medical Center, ended my yearly check-up with a slight deviation from the routine, "The results are fine. See you next year!" remarks.

This time, Dr. Davison sat me down and said, "Hmmm. The results are fine. Thanks for coming in. But, ya know... Your heart valve may need to be replaced someday. I'm sure it won't be for another thirty or forty years... But, for now, I'd like you to start taking this medication. It might help delay any surgical procedure."

Thinking back on that conversation, I am amazed at how I reacted to Dr. Davison's observations. Perhaps I was afraid. Perhaps I didn't trust him. Perhaps I didn't care about what might happen in thirty or forty years.

That said, I paid Dr. Davison's counsel no attention. I didn't take the medication. And, I acted out against him.

"What does he know?" I thought to myself, "The guy got his medical degree from Buenos Aires University in Argentina. Back in 1963."

I didn't return for a yearly echocardiogram for five years after that. Little did I know, my valve was slowly wearing down. And, little did I know, Dr. Davison would be right. I would need to have my valve replaced.

However, I would need my valve replaced twenty to thirty years before he estimated.

Europe And Heart Valve Stress Do Not Mix

The day after Dr. Bad Bedside Manner informed me that I was in need of a new heart valve, I left the United States for a two-week business trip through Europe.

Needless to say, that was a very bad decision.

After traveling through four countries during my first week in Europe, I collapsed when I reached Amsterdam on a Friday night. The stress generated by my troubled heart triggered both emotional and physical problems.

I suffered from chest pains and chest cramps. I could not eat. I could not sleep.

My subconscious was terrorizing my conscious. I was scared, nervous, confused and I was thousands of miles from home. After sharing my condition with my brother on the phone, my mother called me minutes later pleading, "Adam come home! Come home now! Please!"

That Saturday, at one o'clock in the morning, I was examined by the hotel doctor at Le Merige Hotel in Amsterdam. Luckily, my vital signs were normal. My symptoms, the doctor told me, were potentially caused from a mild panic attack not a decompensating heart.

Once the doctor left my hotel room, I immediately called the airlines and rerouted my ticket. I would be returning home the next day. My first plane left in six hours. I began packing immediately.

Thankfully, the doctor gave me two valium to calm my nerves.

Coming Home Early...

There are no words to describe my return home to Los Angeles. I was so thankful to be home. I was happy to see Robyn and my family. I was relieved. I was comfortable again.

I took a few days off from work. My insomnia lessened and I was able to regain some peace of mind.

It didn't take long, however, for me to face the reality of my medical situation.

Yes. I was home. Yes. I was happy. But, I was also in need of a heart valve replacement.

I took action. My heart needed to be fixed. It was now time to learn more about my heart valve disorder and plan the next steps.

Heart Valve Surgery Patient Success Story:
Andy Karplus and Clay Donne

(Source: Edwards LifeSciences)

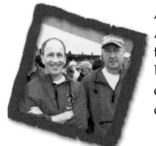 Andy Karplus and Clay Donne make unlikely friends. Andy, 46 years old and better known as Professor Karplus to his students, teaches biochemistry at Oregon State University. 54-year-old Clay, represents a large Oregon company that manufactures wood products for the construction industry.

A shocking discovery brought the two men together when both of them learned they were suffering from life-threatening heart valve disease.

In Clay's case, it was his body that told him he was in trouble. Says Clay, "The defining point was body-surfing in Hawaii and getting to the beach, and standing there in six inches of water, not being able to move."

For Andy, it was a doctor who caught the problem before it was too late. Andy remarks, "I don't like to think about what it would have meant in my case if I hadn't happened to have a physician who noticed the heart murmur, because I could have already had heart failure, that's how bad the leak was."

Within months, Andy and Clay each underwent open-heart surgery to replace their diseased aortic valves. Clay had his surgery performed by Dr. Albert Starr, while Andy's was done by Dr. Anthony Furnary, both at the St. Vincent's Hospital in Portland. Both men received the Carpentier-Edwards PERIMOUNT valve.

"The Edwards valve has given me total freedom and really no limits," says Andy. "I don't even think about the fact that I have an artificial valve in me. That's how free I am."

With hearts good as new, Clay and Andy took on the biggest physical challenge of their lives. Andy, Clay, and ten other open-heart surgery survivors put their hearts and bodies to the test as they participated in the world's largest and longest relay race. **Because the team is composed of all open-heart surgery survivors, they nicknamed themselves "Scar Trek."**

Team Scar Trek took to the pavement in Oregon's famous Hood-to-Coast relay, beginning at the top of Oregon's Mt. Hood. Each team member ran a portion of the 197-mile long course, and at the end of 32 non-stop hours, the team celebrated its special bond and triumph together at the finish in Seaside, Oregon.

Says Clay, "If we hadn't had the Edwards valve, there is no way in the world we could accomplish this kind of task, this race. No way in the world."

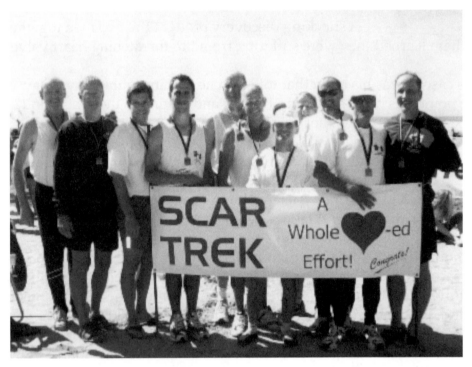

(Source: Andrew Karplus)

3

Your Heart And Your Heart Valves

....

In this chapter, you will:
- Learn about the structure of your *heart* and your *heart valves*.
- Be advised to get a *second opinion*.
- Better understand the different types of valve disorders and symptoms.

....

I don't know about you, but when my cardiologist diagnosed my valve disorder, I only *really* understood about ten percent of the medical terms he used during that conversation. It was like Dr. Bad Bedside Manner was speaking the foreign language of Urdu. I had no idea what *stenosis*, *regurgitation* or *calcification* meant.

To remedy my confusion, I began researching the anatomy of my heart and my heart valves. I really wanted to understand what was wrong. Plus, I wanted to know how surgery was going to make it right.

I also took the time to get a second opinion from a different cardiologist. I highly encourage you to do the same thing. Get a second everything! A second echocardiogram... A second EKG.

I recently conducted a survey of many heart valve surgery patients. One of the questions I asked them was, "Did you get a second opinion to confirm your heart valve defect or disease?" I was shocked when I learned the results. While the majority of patients responded *yes* to that question, more than 35% of the respondents answered *no*!

Did You Get A Second Opinion To Confirm Your Valve Disease Or Defect?
(Source: www.Heart-Valve-Surgery.com)

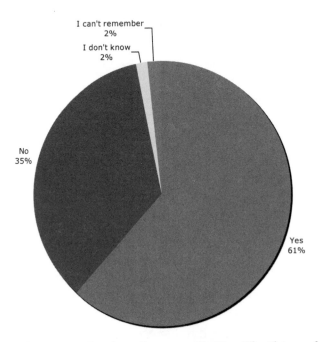

I'll never forget what happened when I met with Dr. Chaikin, a highly regarded cardiologist in Los Angeles, for my second opinion. Unlike most doctors, Dr. Chaikin was physically present during my echocardiogram. He stood next to the technician and observed the ultrasonic images which appeared on the monitor.

"Yep! Right there!" Dr. Chaikin pointed to the monitor and queried the technician, "Let's see that. What is the measurement?"

Dr. Chaikin nodded and asked again, "Ah-huh! And what about that right there? What's that measurement?"

"Hmmmmm. That's enough," he concluded the echo and thanked the technician for her help.

Dr. Chaikin then grabbed a towel and wiped the gel off my bare chest. The lights in the room came back on.

"Well," Dr. Chaikin said.

He then took a sizeable breath and offered his medical opinion. "It is time Adam," he said, "There is severe stenosis and regurgitation in the valve. The heart is dilated. And, I would not wait on this. Not more than thirty days."

His urgency was apparent as he transitioned the conversation to the next step, "I know a great surgeon that is just a few miles from here. Dr. Trento is a magician. I've personally seen him operate."

Dr. Chaikin must have seen the disappointment in my eyes as tears fluttered across my eyelids. He then put his hand on my shoulder and said, "Don't worry. You are going to do just fine. The heart is an amazing muscle."

In that moment, I really did not want to hear about how *amazing* the heart was. If my heart was so amazing, why was it failing me?

(So you know, I am writing these words one year after my surgery. I now agree with Dr. Chaikin. The heart is an amazing muscle. Let us now learn a little bit more about it.)

Your Amazing Heart

Your heart is a blood-pumping machine. According to The Cleveland Clinic, your heart will beat approximately 2.5 billion times during your lifetime. That said, on any given day, your heart will beat up to 100,000 times.

The Texas Heart Institute suggests that most hearts can pump up to 2,000 gallons of blood during each twenty-four hour period.

While most people believe that the human heart is shaped like the image on a common Valentine's Day card, this is actually an incorrect visualization of the cardiac muscle.

According to the National Heart Lung and Blood Institute, "The heart is shaped like an upside-down pear."

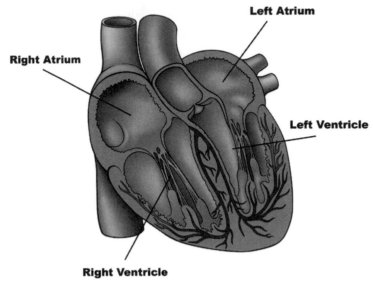

Cavities of the Heart

The human heart is made of a special kind of muscle called myocardium and is enclosed in a double-layered, membranous sac called a pericardium.

A wall of muscle (the septum) divides the heart into two cavities: the left cavity pumps blood throughout the body, while the right cavity pumps blood only through the lungs.

As shown on the figure, there are four cavities in the heart. The two upper chambers of the heart are called atrium, the bottom chambers are called ventricles. **A valve connects each atrium to the ventricle below.**

The right side of the heart receives deoxygenated blood from all parts of the body except for the lungs. The left side of the heart receives oxygenated blood from the lungs and pumps it to the rest of the body.

Other interesting facts about the heart include:

- On average, the heart contracts and relaxes about 70 to 80 times per minute without you ever having to think about it. This is called your heartbeat.

- As the cardiac muscle contracts it pushes blood through the chambers and into the vessels. Nerves connected to the heart regulate the speed with which the muscle contracts. When you run, your heart pumps more quickly. When you sleep, your heart pumps more slowly.

- Considering how much work it has to do, the heart is surprisingly small. The average adult heart is about the size of a clenched fist and weighs around 11 ounces.

- Located in the middle of the chest behind the breastbone, between the lungs, the heart rests in a moistened chamber called the pericardial cavity which is surrounded by the ribcage. The diaphragm, a tough layer of muscle, lies below. As a result, the heart is well protected.

The Anatomy Of Your Four Heart Valves

As you read above, your heart has four chambers. The upper two chambers are atria. The lower two chambers are ventricles. Blood is pumped through the chambers, aided by your four heart valves. There are four different valves in your heart. They are most commonly known as *the aortic valve, the pulmonary valve, the tricuspid valve and the mitral valve.*

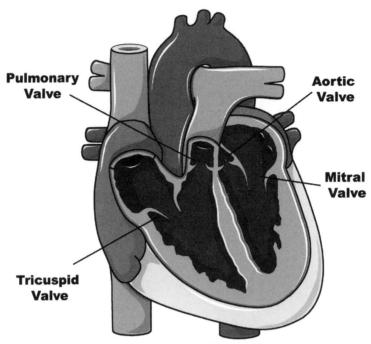

Pulmonary Valve

Aortic Valve

Mitral Valve

Tricuspid Valve

Valves of the Heart (Source: Servier International)

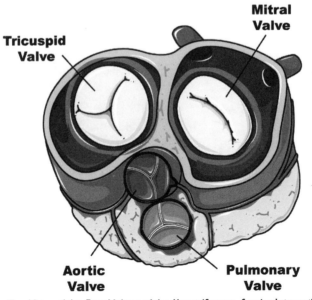

Tricuspid Valve

Mitral Valve

Aortic Valve

Pulmonary Valve

Top View of the Four Valves of the Heart (Source: Servier International)

What Do Your Valves Do?

Your heart valves have a very simple job. They evolved to keep blood flowing in one direction through your heart. Your valves open to let blood flow through and then close to prevent blood from flowing back.

In some ways, your heart valves are very similar to the plumbing valves in your home, which regulate the movement of water through your shower, toilet, sink, washer and sprinklers.

When a valve closes, flaps of tissue on the valve close tightly together to create a seal. These flaps of tissue are called *leaflets*. When working properly, the heart valves open and close fully so that blood keeps moving in one direction at all times.

The Different Types Of Valves

Blood flows through each valve one time on its way through your heart. The four valves can be grouped by their job:

- The tricuspid and mitral valve control blood flow between your heart's upper and lower chambers.

- The aortic and pulmonary valves control blood flow out of your heart.

Valve Problems, Disorders And Abnormalities

Like most physical things in life (e.g. your car or your phone), problems can occur with your heart valves. Sometimes, a person can be born with an abnormal heart valve, also known as a *congenital heart defect*. Other people may experience valve damage due to infections, rheumatic fever and changes in valve structure due to the aging process.

The Cardiac Cycle
How Blood Flows Through The Heart

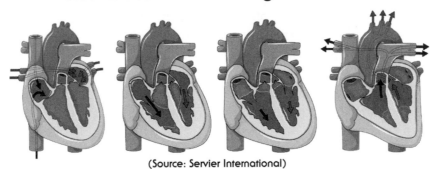

(Source: Servier International)

While it is true that valve problems typically impact seniors, many different age groups require medical procedures to address cardiac problems that result from valve dysfunction including newborns and adolescents.

I recently conducted an online survey to learn more about the age groups which experience heart valve operations. It was interesting to see that respondents aged 31-45 were just as prevalent (38%) as the 46-60 age group (38%).

What Was Your Age At The Time Of Your Heart Valve Surgery?
(Source: www.Heart-Valve-Surgery.com)

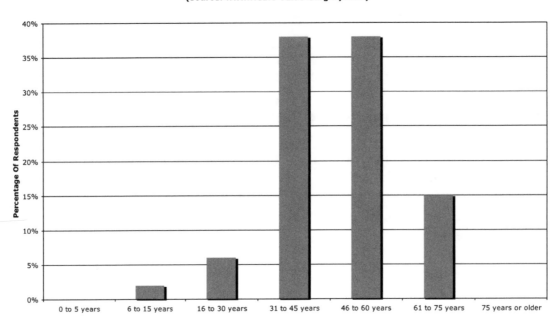

One of the common questions I receive from patients over eighty years of age is, **"Am I too old for heart valve surgery?"** Recently, some interesting data has been published about this exact topic - valve surgery in patients over eighty years old.

Dr. Farzan Filsoufi and his colleagues from the Mount Sinai School of Medicine in New York City found that patients 80 years of age or older who underwent aortic valve replacement fared nearly as well as younger patients. The study, published in *The Journal of the American Geriatrics Society*, reviewed the records of 1,308 consecutive patients who underwent the procedure at Mount Sinai between 1998 and 2006. Of these patients, 17.6 percent were 80 or older. The report found that older patients were no more likely to die in the hospital than the younger patients.

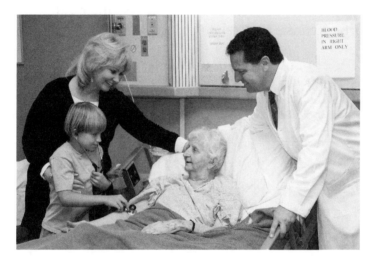

The real good news of the report? About two thirds of the oldest patients lived for at least 5 years after the operation, a rate of survival comparable to people of the same age in the general population. Dr. Filsoufi believes that the advances in cardiac surgery technology is the key reason for the positive findings of the study.

What is a defective heart valve?

Most problems associated with valve damage are associated with the opening and the closing of the valve. *Remember, a properly functioning heart valve regulates the flow of blood in one direction.* If a valve doesn't open all the way, less blood moves through to the next chamber. If a valve doesn't close tightly, blood may leak backward.

These problems may impact the heart and force it to work harder to pump the same amount of blood. Therefore, a defective heart valve typically results from these two problems:

Problems opening. *Stenosis* occurs when a valve fails to open fully. Valves that are stenotic may be hardened or stiff with calcium deposits or scarring. Or, in some congenital cases, aortic valves may have only two leaflets (bicuspid) while most normal valves have three leaflets (tricuspid). Ultimately, stenotic valves are hard to push open. This is problematic because blood has to flow through a smaller opening. So, less blood advances during each heartbeat.

The American Heart Association has developed specific guidelines which describe the severity of aortic stenosis as it relates to valve gradient, area and velocity.

Classification of Aortic Stenosis

Severity	Valve Area (cm²)	Maximum Aortic Velocity (m/sec)	Mean Pressure Gradient (mmHg)
Mild	1.5 - 2.0	2.5 - 3.0	< 25
Moderate	1.0 - 1.5	3.0 - 4.0	25 - 40
Severe	0.6 - 1.0	> 4.0	> 40
Critical	< 0.6	—	—

(Source: The Cleveland Clinic)

- *Gradient.* A normal aortic valve has no gradient. If the aortic valve mean gradient is <25 mm Hg, the stenosis is mild; if the mean gradient is between 25 mm Hg and 40 mm Hg, the stenosis is moderate; and, if the mean gradient is >40 mm Hg, the stenosis is severe.

- *Valve Area.* A normal aortic valve area is >2 cm². If the valve area is between 1.5 and 2.0 cm², the stenosis is mild; if the valve area is between 1.0 and 1.5 cm², the stenosis is moderate; if the valve area is between 0.6 and 1.0 cm², the stenosis is moderate-to-severe; and, areas less than 0.6 cm² constitute severe aortic stenosis.

- *Aortic Velocity.* As for velocity, mild stenosis is between 2.5 and 3.0 m/sec; moderate stenosis is between 3.0 and 4.0 m/sec and severe stenosis is >4.0 m/sec.

Problems closing. Insufficient blood flow (also called *regurgitation*) results when the valve fails to close tightly. A valve with regurgitation may result from its physical structure being loose or torn. This is problematic because blood may leak backwards through the valve. The heart then has to work harder to *re-pump* the blood through the heart.

As with stenosis, there are guidelines which help classify heart valves with regurgitation. According to Dr. David Adams' excellent website, www. mitralvalverepair.org, the two main determinants in quantifying mitral regurgitation are regurgitation volume and effective regurgitant orifice.

Classification of Mitral Regurgitation		
MR grade	Rvol (ml)	ERO (mm²)
Mild	< 30	< 20
Moderate	30 - 59	20 - 39
Severe	≥ 60	≥ 40

(Source: Dr. David Adams, Mount Sinai Hospital)

Regurgitation volume (RVOL) is the difference between the mitral and aortic stroke volumes. A mitral valve with a RVOL less than 30 ml is mild; a RVOL between 30-39 ml is moderate; and a RVOL greater than 60 is severe.

Effective regurgitant orifice (ERO) is the ratio of regurgitant volume to regurgitant time velocity integral. If the ERO of a mitral valve is less than 20 mm^2, it is mild; an ERO of 20-39 mm^2 is moderate; and, an ERO greater than 40 mm^2 is severe.

What Are The Common Symptoms Associated With Damaged Heart Valves?

There are a number of common symptoms among individuals with heart valve disorders. As we just learned, these symptoms typically result from either heart valve stenosis or regurgitation. If the narrowing (stenosis) is severe - the heart has to pump harder to get blood past the narrowing. If the leak is severe (regurgitation) - the heart has to pump harder to advance the blood that leaks backwards.

In both cases, this can put additional strain on the heart. There may be an increase in pressure behind the affected valve. This pressure can cause blood and fluid to build up in the lungs or lower part of the body (depending on which valve is affected).

The Cleveland Clinic and The Mayo Clinic suggest there are many symptoms which may result from heart valve disorders including, but not limited to:

- Shortness of breath, especially with exertion or when you lie down
- Fatigue, especially during times of increased activity
- Cough, especially at night or when lying down
- Heart palpitations — sensations of a rapid, fluttering heartbeat
- Swollen feet or ankles
- Heart murmur
- Excessive urination
- Chest pain (angina) or tightness
- Feeling faint or fainting with exertion
- Dizziness

As a result, various complications may develop, depending on the valve affected and the severity of the problem.

The Steps To Identifying Heart Valve Disorders

Heart valve disease can be identified in several ways. First, a doctor can simply listen to your heart with a stethoscope. This is usually the first step in diagnosing heart valve disease. A heart murmur (abnormal sounds in the heart due to turbulent blood flow) can often indicate valve regurgitation.

To better diagnose valve disease and valve damage, physicians may use the following diagnostic procedures:

- **Electrocardiogram (ECG or EKG)** - a test that records the electrical activity of the heart, shows abnormal rhythms (arrhythmias or dysrhythmias), and detects heart muscle damage.

- **Chest x-ray** - a diagnostic test which uses invisible electromagnetic energy beams to produce images of internal tissues, bones, and organs onto film. An x-ray can show enlargement in any area of the heart.

· **Cardiac catheterization** - this diagnostic procedure involves a tiny, hollow tube (catheter) being inserted into an artery leading to the heart in order to image the heart and blood vessels. This procedure is helpful in determining the type and extent of valve blockage.

· **Echocardiogram** – a diagnostic test that uses sound waves that bounce off the heart, creating a graphic image of the movement of the heart structures.

· **Transesophageal echocardiogram (TEE)** - a transesophageal echo uses an ultrasound transducer that is positioned on an endoscope and guided down the patient's throat into the esophagus (the "food pipe" leading from the mouth into the stomach). The TEE test provides a close look at the heart's valves and chambers, without interference from the ribs or lungs. TEE is often used when the results from standard echo tests are not sufficient, or when your doctor wants a closer look at your heart, according to The Cleveland Clinic.

· **Radionuclide scans** - these scans use radioactive imaging to view blood flow, internal organ structure, and organ function.

· **Magnetic resonance imaging (MRI)** - a diagnostic procedure that uses a combination of large magnets, radiofrequencies, and a computer to produce detailed images of organs and structures within the body.

My Personal Story With Heart Valve Diagnosis And Symptoms

As you read in my story, I had severe aortic stenosis and regurgitation when I learned that I needed a heart valve replacement. Both of my cardiologists confirmed the severity of the defect using an echocardiogram.

The interesting element of my diagnosis was that I had *almost no symptoms* of heart valve disease. Of the ten symptoms listed above, I really only experienced one symptom which led me to seek medical help. However, please note that even though I was mostly asymptomatic my heart was already enlarged and beginning to show signs of damage.

As many patients are asymptomatic, I highly encourage you to visit your doctor if you are experiencing any of the symptoms above.

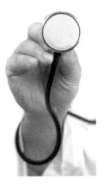

Did You Know?

When you listen to your heartbeat through a stethoscope, you hear the sound of your heart valves closing. That sound is typically known as a "lubb-dubb".

Although your heart has four valves, the valves open and close two at a time. That's why you hear only two thumps (one "lubb-dubb") per heartbeat.

"Can Medication Treat My Heart Valve Disease?" Asks Jimmy
Adam's Heart Valve Surgery Blog Excerpt - Posted On July 6, 2009

Jimmy just sent me a great question about the use of medications to treat heart valve disease.

He writes, "Adam - On Friday, I was diagnosed with mitral valve prolapse. I've been short of breath for sometime but had no idea it was due to a heart valve problem. My cardiologist thinks I need a valve replacement within the next six months. I'm shocked and in 'Why Me?' mode right now. Given my disbelief, I'm curious to know if there are any medications that can treat heart valve disease? As you may have guessed, I'm not very excited about open heart surgery. Any thoughts? Thanks, Jimmy"

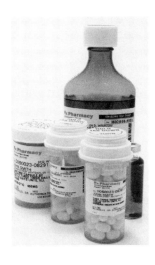

I have to admit… Jimmy's question just brought back a memory. It was November, 2005 when my cardiologist informed that I needed heart valve replacement surgery.

I'll never forget that uncomfortable moment.

I'll also never forget one of the first questions I asked the cardiologist, *"Can we treat this with medication?"*

Dr. Bad Bedside Manner snipped back at me, "Not at this point. Your valve is both stenotic and suffering from regurgitation. Medication won't make any difference. You need a valve replacement. Any other questions?"

As noted earlier, my bicuspid aortic valve was in very bad shape and needed to be replaced. However, you should know that if you are diagnosed with mild or moderate forms of heart valve disease, medication may be prescribed by your doctor to help relieve symptoms and decrease the risk of further damage to your heart.

Some of the medications that may be prescribed to help manage heart valve disorders are:

- ACE inhibitors
- Beta-blockers
- Diuretics / water pills
- Vasodilators

Although helpful, these medications will not reverse pre-existing damage to your heart valves.

As the Mayo Clinic reports, "Medications can help reduce the heart's workload and regulate its rhythm. In some cases, medication can slow progressive mitral valve disease. However, no medications can cure heart valve disease."

You should know that valvular damage can progress even if the patient is using the above-referenced medications. In those situations, the patient typically requires surgical treatment in the form of heart valve repair or heart valve replacement surgery.

I hope this helps you better understand how medications are used to help, but not reverse, heart valve disease.

Keep on tickin!

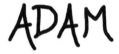

4

A Guardian Angel Appears At Dinner

By the time Dr. Chaikin confirmed I would need heart valve surgery, it was late on a Wednesday evening. Luckily, my mom, Donna, accompanied me to that appointment.

My mom immediately hugged me as we left the medical office and proceeded down the hallway to the elevator shaft.

 If possible, I highly encourage you to go to all major doctor and hospital visits with a friend or family member. You may want or need their support.

With Dr. Chaikin's second opinion, there was no longer a gray zone for me to hide. I had no logical option but to have the operation.

In that moment, I remember the optimist in me rising up.

"Settle down Adam," I thought to myself, "This is going to be just fine. You will be okay."

Perhaps this was my coping mechanism. Perhaps, I immediately glorified the positive because the negative was filled with potential mortality. And, between you and me, I was not ready to die just yet.

So, as my mom and I left Dr. Chaikin's office, we did not cry. We did not lash out against the world. We did not manifest anger. We did not feel pity. We did not soak each other in sorrow.

Rather, we did what any other mother and son would do at seven o'clock on a

Wednesday night. We went to Louise's Tratorria on Pico Boulevard for some good Italian food. Robyn, my wife, met us shortly thereafter. All of us had a glass of red wine and feasted on the best eggplant parmesan in Los Angeles.

As I remember it, we spoke very little about Dr. Chaikin or my heart during the dinner.

However, as we were finishing up our second glass of Pinot Noir, an elderly man dressed in jeans and a nice sweater approached our table.

The man looked at me and said, "I'm sorry to interrupt. But, I couldn't help but overhear your conversation. I was sitting with my wife right over there."

He pointed to a table behind us with no one in it.

"I want you to know something," the sweet man said in a very calming voice, "You are going to be just fine."

I squinted in curiosity and disbelief. He continued, "I have had my heart operated on twice." He simultaneously pointed to his chest with both hands.

"Three years ago, my heart was taken out of my body and fixed," he shared.

"Look at me now! I'm doing great! Don't you worry about a thing!" he exclaimed.

A second later, the man was gone.

We did not exchange names.

I did not have time to ask him any questions.

The conversation ended as soon as it started.

Robyn, my mom and I were in shock.

We couldn't process what had just happened.

Then, I realized what had just happened.

I had encountered a guardian angel.

He said that I would be fine.

I trusted him.

It was now time to determine my surgical options and find a surgeon.

chapter

5

Heart Valve Surgery Options

....

In this chapter, you will:
- Learn about heart valve repair surgeries.
- Learn about heart valve replacement procedures.
- Understand the different kinds of valve replacements – mechanical and tissue valves.
- Read about my heart valve surgery – *The Ross Procedure*.

....

Following the conversation with my guardian angel, I was ready to take the next steps. I knew I had to find a heart surgeon but I also wanted to learn more about heart valve surgery.

I went scouring the Internet looking for different options for people with defective valves. I learned that there were two key forms of heart valve surgery – valve repair and valve replacement.

Heart Valve Repair Surgery

Heart valve repair surgery involves a procedure to fix your heart valve, as opposed to replacing it with a mechanical or tissue valve. Different techniques can be used to repair a heart valve depending upon the problem.

The objectives of heart valve repair are:

- Reshaping of the valve by removing excess valve tissue.
- Adding support to the valve ring by adding tissue or a collarlike structure around the base of the valve.

- Attaching the valve to nearby heart cordlike tissues (chordal transposition).

The Cleveland Clinic suggests that the advantages of heart valve repair are lower risk of infection, decreased need for life-long blood thinner medication, and preserved heart muscle strength. The mitral valve is the most commonly repaired valve, but the aortic and tricuspid valves may also need repair procedures.

According to The Texas Heart Institute, the most common heart valve repair procedures include:

- *Commissurotomy,* which is used for narrowed valves, where the leaflets are thickened and perhaps stuck together. The surgeon opens the valve by cutting the points where the leaflets meet.

- *Valvuloplasty,* which strengthens the leaflets to provide more support and to let the valve close tightly. This support comes from a ring-like device that surgeons attach around the outside of the valve opening.

- *Reshaping,* where the surgeon cuts out a section of a leaflet. Once the leaflet is sewn back together, the valve can close properly.

- *Decalcification,* which removes calcium buildup from the leaflets. Once the calcium is removed, the leaflets can close properly.

- *Repair of structural support,* which replaces or shortens the cords that give the valves support. When the cords are the right length, the valve can close properly.

- *Patching,* where the surgeon covers holes or tears in the leaflets with a tissue patch.

It is important to note that some surgeons are performing heart valve repairs through *minimally invasive approaches*. One form of non-invasive valve repair uses a three-inch keyhole incision on the side of the chest. This approach avoids a major incision in the breastbone and allows patients to return to work and everyday activity sooner after surgery.

Mitral valve repair surgery is also being done with the help of robotic machines which minimize trauma to the body. The leading device for robotic heart valve repair surgery is the *da Vinci Surgical System*.

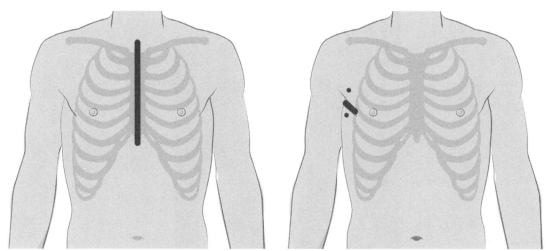

Incision Comparison: Open Heart versus da Vinci Robot
(Source: Intuitive Surgical)

Unlike traditional open heart procedures, your surgeon can use the *da Vinci* robot to fix the mitral valve with a few small incisions (as shown above). Some surgeons, including Dr. Randolph Chitwood of the East Carolina Heart Institute, have performed over 400 mitral valve repair surgeries using robotic machines.

Finally, as referenced in the opening of this book, several new technologies are being developed to treat heart valves without any formal incision to the sternum.

For example, percutaneous mitral valve repair can be performed by physicians in a catheterization laboratory. During this procedure, the heart beats normally. Therefore, a heart-lung bypass machine is not required. In addition to improving blood flow through the heart, the procedure may also relieve symptoms such as fatigue and shortness of breath that often affect patients with mitral regurgitation.

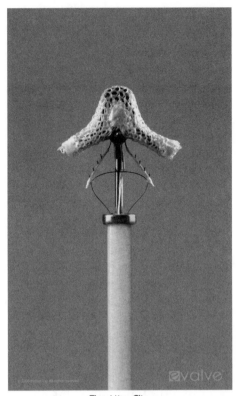

The MitraClip
(Source: Abbott Laboratories)

One such catheter-based technology for mitral valve repair is the MitraClip by Abbott Laboratories. The MitraClip has already received a CE mark in Europe and reports suggest that this non-invasive approach could be approved by the FDA in the United States within the next few years.

Heart Valve Replacement Surgery

Heart valve replacement surgery is required for patients with heart valves that are severely damaged beyond surgical repair. Valve replacement procedures are most often used to treat aortic valves and severely damaged mitral valves.

There are two common kinds of valves used for valve replacement surgeries — mechanical and biological valves.

Mitral Valve Replacement With
Tissue or Mechanical Valve Option

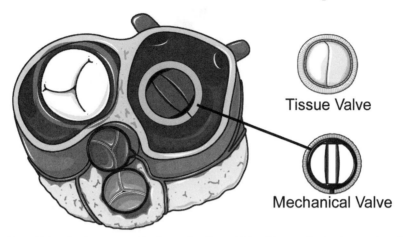

Tissue Valve

Mechanical Valve

Heart Valve Replacement - Mechanical or Tissue Valve (Source: Servier International)

Mechanical Valve Replacements

Mechanical valves, also known as artificial valves, are carefully designed to mimic the human heart valve. They have a ring, like your own natural heart valve, to support its leaflets. And, like your own heart valve, the mechanical valve opens and closes with each heartbeat, permitting proper blood flow through the heart.

Mechanical valves are made from materials such as plastic, carbon, or metal. Therefore, mechanical valves are strong and can last more than thirty years. During my research for this book, I spoke with several patients that had mechanical valves implanted in the 1970's. Yes... The 1970's!

However, because blood tends to stick to mechanical valve materials inside the body, it is necessary to protect the patient from blood clots. To prevent any blood clots from developing on the valve, patients are typically required to take anticoagulation medicine (blood thinners) daily.

The dosage of this anticoagulant, usually Coumadin, is different for each person. That said, patients are monitored to make sure they are on the correct dosage.

Regular blood tests will be performed at the physician's office, an anticoagulation clinic, or at home with a specialized testing kit.

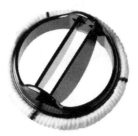

The St. Jude Medical Regent Mechanical Heart Valve
(Source: St. Jude Medical)

During my research for this book, I asked several patients, *"What is life like on Coumadin?"* Responses to that question are provided below:

- Jonathan said, "I am a 29 year old male and have been on Coumadin since 2002 for a mechanical aortic valve replacement. My experience has been mostly positive. Activity wise, I am doing everything I have enjoyed doing most of my life - surfing, basketball, etc. I do bruise a little easier these days and you need to be careful about head injuries, but really the worse thing about Coumadin is needing to go to the clinic to get blood drawn every 2-3 weeks. Besides that, life isn't that much different on Coumadin and it's really not a big deal. I hope this helps!"

- Lee said, "I have been on Coumadin since I had my aortic valve replaced with a St. Jude valve on December 4, 2008. I have not had any problems with bleeding or bruising that I was warned about from my doctor. The only problem was remembering to take my dosage every day. But with an alarm to remind me, that is not a problem anymore. For anybody trying to decide on a mechanical or tissue valve, do not let the Coumadin keep you from choosing a mechanical valve.

- Kemal said, "Once you get used to it, life on Coumadin is not much different. I suggest ordering a home-test device for PT/INR testing."

To read 30 more responses to the question, "What is life like on Coumadin?", please visit http://www.heart-valve-surgery.com/2009/03/27/what-is-life-like-on-coumadin/.

You should also know that some mechanical valve replacement devices are being investigated for lower dosages of anticoagulation therapy. For example, the On-X prosthetic heart valve replacement is a pure carbon bi-leaflet heart valve prosthesis. One of the most interesting attractions of the On-X valve is the fact that in January, 2006, the FDA approved the first-and-only IDE (Investigational Device Exemption) lowered anticoagulation trial for a mechanical valve to be conducted at 40 sites in the United States.

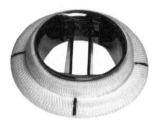

On-X Mitral Valve Replacement
(Source: ON-X Life Technologies)

The Clicking Noise. By design, most mechanical valves make a closing sound (or click) as they open and close. This may be important to you if you are faced with heart valve replacement and your cardiac surgeon has determined you are a candidate for a mechanical valve. The type of mechanical valve, its size, and the patient's body height and weight are all factors in the intensity of noise heard. Since the design and closing mechanisms are unique to each mechanical valve, some designs are more likely to produce more noticeable sounds than others.

During an interview with a recent heart valve replacement patient, Susan said, "I just turned 50, and it has only been 7 weeks since my valve replacement surgery. I got a St. Jude valve. I do hear a small clicking noise when it is really quiet and I am lying on my back. It usually doesn't bother me. But if it does, I roll on my right side and it disappears. No one else in my family can hear it click."

Biological Valve Replacements

There are a variety of biological alternatives for heart valve replacements. However, most tissue valves are made from pigs and cows (called a *xenograft*). Once the valve structure / tissue is removed from the animal, it is chemically treated and prepared for human use.

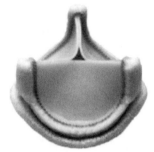

Carpentier-Edwards® PERIMOUNT Magna® Valve Made from Bovine Pericardial Tissue
(Source: Edwards Lifesciences)

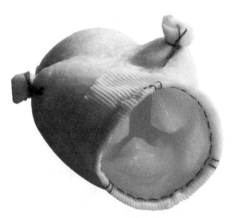

Medtronic Freestyle Aortic Root Bioprosthesis
(Source: Medtronic)

A *homograft* or *allograft* is a human valve obtained from a human donor. This type of valve is particularly beneficial for pregnant women and children, because it does not require long-term anticoagulation therapy.

Sometimes, a patient's own tissue can be used for valve replacement (called an *autograft*) in a valve replacement procedure known as the *Ross Procedure*.

The key advantage of a biological valve is that it has a reduced risk of blood clots forming on the valve. Therefore, the patient is not required to take an anticoagulant (e.g. Coumadin). However, the key disadvantage of biological valves is that they have limited durability as compared with mechanical valves.

Mechanical Or Biological Heart Valves?

There are trade-offs to choosing a mechanical or a biological heart valve replacement. The main trade-off between mechanical and tissue valves is durability versus risk of blood clots. A mechanical valve may last 20 to 30 years, while a tissue valve may last about 10 to 15 years. However, the risk of blood clotting is higher with a mechanical valve. Blood clots can cause a heart attack or stroke.

In my opinion, this is one of the toughest decisions you will make if you are preparing for heart valve replacement surgery. Ultimately, you should discuss this valve choice (at length) with your surgeon and your family.

Minimally Invasive Approaches To Heart Valve Replacement

Many surgeons, cardiologists and heart valve manufacturers are currently working on minimally invasive approaches to heart valve replacement. Similar to minimally invasive heart valve repair procedures, the key patient benefits include less pain, shorter hospital stay and accelerated recovery.

The main types of minimally invasive heart valve replacement procedures include mini-sternotomy, mini-thoracotomy and catheter-based approaches.

According to Brigham & Women's Cardiovascular Center, a **mini-sternotomy** can be performed through very small incisions (3 inches) compared with those used in conventional surgery.

- Mini-sternotomy for aortic valve replacement incisions are performed through an upper mini-sternotomy, in which an incision is made from the sternal notch to the third intercostal space.

- Mini-sternotomy for mitral valve replacement incisions are performed through a lower mini-sternotomy, in which a 6-8 cm incision is made at the lower end of the sternum upward to the second intercostal space and extending into the interspace on the right.

As to the clinical use of mini-sternotomy, Dr. Eric Roselli, cardiac surgeon at The Cleveland Clinic noted, "Almost all isolated first time aortic valves get a mini-sternotomy in my practice and I believe that's true for my colleagues as well."

Specific to **mini-thoracotomy** for valve replacement, Columbia University Medical Center suggests that a mini-thoracotomy uses a 2-inch incision made between the ribs.

Commenting on his recent aortic valve replacement, Jim Englemann noted, "Adam - I had the minimally invasive surgery through a mini-thoracotomy on January 19, 2009. I really had faith in my surgeon. I believed he had a thorough process just in case there were any problems. My medical team did not have to break the sternum. Instead they entered my chest from above the heart. The operation, which was 7.5 hours, went well."

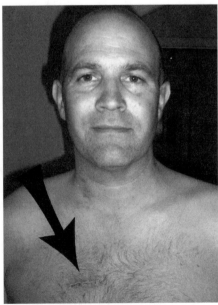

Patient Scar After Mini-Thoracotomy
(Source: Jim Engelmann)

Finally, one of the most exciting, minimally invasive surgical approaches being developed, tested and evaluated for patients requiring heart valve replacement surgery is the use of biological valve replacements delivered through a catheter.

For example, the Edwards SAPIEN valve is an investigational device being evaluated in the treatment of patients with severe aortic stenosis who are considered to be high-risk or non-operable for conventional open-heart valve replacement surgery.

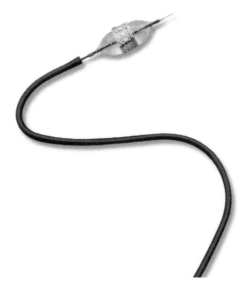

Edwards SAPIEN Valve
(Courtesy: Edwards Lifesciences)

In the first post-commercial study of over 1,000 patients in Europe, clinical data presented about the Edwards SAPIEN valve showed a 30-day survival rate of 93.7% in transfemoral procedures through the femoral artery, and 89.7% in transapical procedures through the left ventricle. These results were better than the predicted surgical survival in the high-risk patient category.

At the present time, the Edwards SAPIEN valve is available in Europe. Reports suggest that this device could receive FDA-approval in the United States within the next few years.

My Heart Valve Surgery Choice... The Ross Procedure

There is another heart valve replacement option to review as we close this chapter. It is known as the Ross Procedure. This was the heart valve surgery I chose. During this operation, the patient's diseased aortic valve is replaced with his or her own pulmonary valve. The pulmonary valve is then replaced with a homograft (a donor human heart valve).

To some extent, a game of musical chairs is played with the patient's pulmonary heart valve. It is moved from the pulmonary position to the aortic position.

Named in honor of its creator, English surgeon Dr. Donald Ross, in the late 1960s, the Ross Procedure is an innovative means of valvular replacement for the aortic valve, particularly in children and patients under 50 years of age. Although cardiac surgeons in the United States began using the procedure in the 1980s, it is still performed only at a very select group of medical centers.

The Ross Procedure has some advantages over traditional procedures:

- **No blood thinners (anticoagulants) are needed after the Ross Procedure.** If the aortic valve is replaced with a mechanical valve, the patient must take anticoagulants for the rest of his or her life. These medications have a small risk of excess bleeding or hemorrhage and the effects of the anticoagulants must be monitored with a blood test every 3 or 4 weeks.

- **No postoperative deterioration by calcification of the valve.** This can be a problem for patients who have their valve replaced with one from an animal (pig or cow). The younger the patient, the less durable the animal valve.

- **The patient's pulmonary valve is typically the right size to replace the aortic valve.**

- **No artificial material is used for the new aortic valve.** This avoids many problems including rejection. Since the new aortic valve is created from the patient's own tissue, the tissue is alive and healthy, instead of being frozen or chemically treated.

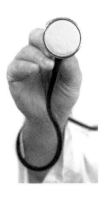

Did You Know?

On April 16, 1997 Arnold Schwarzenegger underwent elective heart surgery to replace a defective, congenital aortic heart valve. Schwarzenegger apparently opted against a mechanical valve and chose a tissue valve because he felt a mechanical valve might limit his physical activity and capacity to exercise.

PART II
PREPARING FOR HEART VALVE SURGERY

chapter

6

Finding The Right Surgeon

In this chapter, you will:
- Develop a strategy for finding the right surgeon.
- Learn the key questions to ask your prospective surgeons.
- Move forward with scheduling your operation.

Now that we understand some of the surgical options available to you, it is time to locate the right surgeon. As you may know, heart surgeons fall into a surgical category known as *cardiothoracic surgeons*. Cardiothoracic surgery is the field of medicine involved in the surgical treatment of diseases affecting organs inside the thorax (your chest), specifically your heart and lungs.

Cardiac surgery and thoracic surgery are separate surgical specialties, but are frequently grouped together as cardiothoracic surgery. Cardiac surgery generally refers to surgery of the heart and vessels, while thoracic surgery generally refers to surgery of the chest other than the heart.

As you may recall, Dr. Chaikin, my second opinion cardiologist, was very quick to refer me to Dr. Trento.

Dr. Alfredo Trento is the Chairman, Division of Cardiothoracic Surgery at Cedars-Sinai Medical Center and holds the Estelle, Abe and Marjorie Sanders Endowed Chair in Cardiac Surgery. Dr. Trento is also Professor of Surgery at the David Geffen School of Medicine at the University of California, Los Angeles (UCLA).

Needless to say, Dr. Trento's credentials are amazing. However, I did not want to rush my surgeon selection. I wanted to find the best surgeon for me.

That said, my family and I began an exhaustive search for the surgeon that would fix my heart. Our search consisted of four, logical actions:

We asked our friends and family! It's quite amazing what happens when your friends and family learn that you are about to have open-heart surgery. All of a sudden, my friends and family became cardiothoracic surgeon gurus. I can not tell you how many people were referring me to well-known surgeons and medical centers. It was very helpful.

We asked medical professionals that we knew! Next, my family reached out to other people in the medical field to see what the professionals thought about the heart surgeon industry. This, I believe, was the most helpful tactic in our surgeon selection process.

Lucky for me, my father, Jerry, is an anesthesiologist here in Los Angeles. He contacted several members of the cardiothoracic community to learn more about the top cardiothoracic surgeons.

In about a week, my dad was able to develop a professional consensus about the best cardiothoracic surgeons in the country. According to his research, Dr. Vaughn Starnes of the University of Southern California Medical Center was the *one*.

In addition, my sister, Monica, talked to several members of the medical community. She also spoke with heart valve surgery patients which she met at an online forum called The Valve Replacement Forum (www.ValveReplacement. com). According to her research, Dr. Chaikin's referral was right on target. Dr. Trento was the *one*.

I also talked to my network of medical professionals including primary physicians, urologists, nurses and sports doctors. According to my research, Dr. Trento was the *one*.

Search the Internet! In this day and age, the Internet is key for researching just about anything, including cardiothoracic surgeons. To learn more about any reputable surgeon, simply type their name into Google (www.google.com) and see what search results appear. I just searched "Alfredo Trento" and "Vaughn Starnes" on Google and clicked on the top search results.

If you don't have a specific surgeon that you are looking for, you may want to start by finding the top medical centers in an area near you. I found the following "Best Hospitals For Heart and Heart Surgery" listing at U.S. News and World Reports website (http://www.usnews.com/usnews/health/best-hospitals/rankings/specihqcard.htm). It's a little overwhelming with data but it might help you.

On the Internet, you will also find a number of referral websites which will help you (i) find heart surgeons, (ii) learn about their capabilities and board certifications, (iii) uncover any misconduct issues and (iv) allow you to compare surgeons against other surgeons.

Most of these services provide some information for free and additional information for a fee. For example, HealthGrades (www.healthgrades.com) will provide you the names of cardiac surgeons in your area at no cost. However, to get detailed analysis about those surgeons, you must pay a fee.

Also, for a listing of heart surgeons in your area, you can visit The CardioThoracic Surgery Network at http://www.ctsnet.org/members/bystate.cfm?ms=Surgeons.

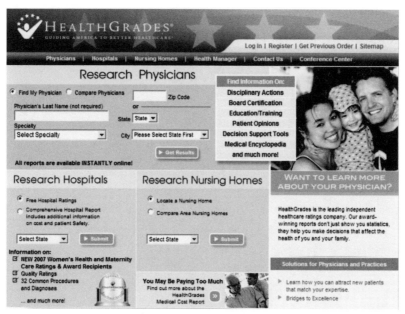

(Source: HealthGrades.com)

The FREE Heart Valve Surgeon Database... Available Now!!!

There is one more, fantastic resource for you to find incredibly great information about heart valve surgeons.

In early 2009, several members from my website, www.Heart-Valve-Surgery.com, discussed the possibility of creating an online, heart valve surgeon database. The idea was to create an easy-to-use surgeon directory with the following objectives:

- To help future patients and caregivers QUICKLY find trusted and reputable heart valve surgeons anywhere in the world.

- To provide surgeon feedback from the PATIENT PERSPECTIVE.

- To offer this information FREE-OF-CHARGE.

Thanks to the support of the heart valve surgery community, this database successfully launched to an overwhelmingly favorable response. Today, the database holds more than 425 surgeon profiles from 25 countries around the world.

That said, I think this online tool might really help you. The database is located at the following address – **http://www.HeartValveSurgeons.com**.

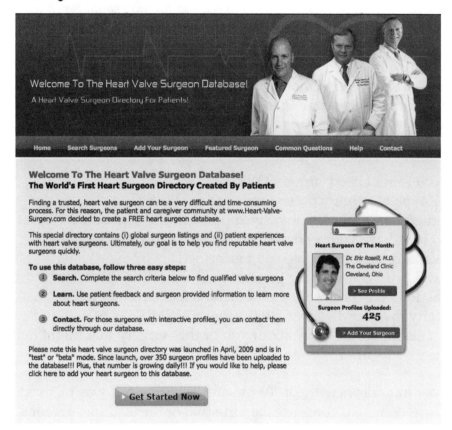

(http://www.HeartValveSurgeons.com)

Interviewing The "Short-List"

When your initial research is complete, you will have a list of potential surgeons. I called this my *short-list*. While I researched several surgeons, the two names that received the most praise were Dr. Trento and Dr. Starnes. My research showed that either surgeon could do the job.

However, I wanted to meet with each surgeon to learn more about them. I also wanted to hear their thoughts about (i) my situation and (ii) the surgical options available to me.

Before my meetings, I prepared a list of questions to review with the doctor. *I also had a copy of my echocardiogram so that each doctor could analyze my condition and provide me their best surgical opinion.*

My question list consisted of mostly open-ended questions. I wanted the doctors to explain their thoughts rather than answer with a simple 'yes' or 'no' response. I just reviewed my notes from my meetings with Dr. Trento and Dr. Starnes. Here are the questions I asked each of the surgeons:

- Do you think I need surgery? Why?
- What type of surgery do you recommend? Why?
- Are there any other less invasive opportunities to consider? What are they?
- How long have you been performing heart valve surgery for?
- How many surgeries have you performed?
- What do you consider my greatest risks from this operation?
- What do you expect is the best outcome from this operation?
- Has anyone ever died from that surgery? Why?
- What else should I know about you or this surgery that might help me make up my mind?

Following my interviews with Dr. Trento and Dr. Starnes, I was relieved. I was happy because there was consensus among two of the leading surgeons. Both men agreed that the Ross Procedure was the best heart valve replacement option for me considering my age and active lifestyle. This was a relief.

My Surgeon Of Choice?

Both surgeons – Dr. Trento and Dr. Starnes – impressed me. Their careers are marked by incredible achievements. I can easily understand why each surgeon was so highly regarded by their peers.

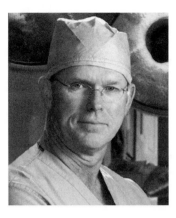

However, I decided to go with my gut. And, my gut told me that Dr. Starnes was the *one*. There were two key reasons why I selected Dr. Starnes.

First, I had a certain feeling of comfort and familiarity with Dr. Starnes that I did not have with Dr. Trento.

As I would later tell my mom, "It felt like our souls knew each other and my soul was willing to trust him with my life."

As you just read, having a high level of personal comfort with the surgeon was critical for me during the interview process. I knew there might be some ups and downs in the hospital and during the recovery from heart valve surgery. Therefore, I wanted to select a surgeon who maintained good bedside manner and communication skills.

Recently, I coordinated an extensive survey with heart valve surgery patients and caregivers. One of the survey questions required respondents to rank their surgeon's bedside manner on a scale of 1 (problematic) to 10 (excellent). I was very pleased to see the majority of respondents (62%) felt their surgeon's bedside manner was *excellent*.

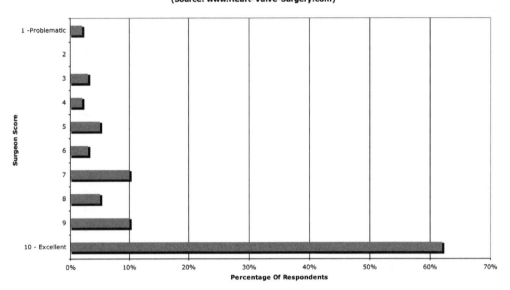

**On A Scale Of 1 (Problematic) To 10 (Excellent),
How Would You Score Your Surgeon's Bedside Manner?
(Source: www.Heart-Valve-Surgery.com)**

Patient Recommended Surgeons

There were a number of cardiac surgeons that were overly praised by their patients in the above-referenced survey and ongoing research. For your review, I have listed those surgeons that are highly regarded by their patients.

- Dr. Kevin Accola (Florida)
- Dr. David Adams (New York)
- Dr. Mark Bleiweis (Florida)
- Dr. Edward Chen (Georgia)
- Dr. Randolph Chitwood (North Carolina)
- Dr. Harry DePan (New York)
- Dr. Ron Elkins (Oklahoma)
- Dr. Jennifer Ellis (Washington, D.C.)
- Dr. Marc Gillinov (Ohio)
- Dr. Vincent Gaudiani (California)
- Dr. Robert Guyton (Georgia)
- Dr. Chiwon Hahn (Virginia)
- Dr. Junaid Khan (California)
- Dr. James Kirklin (Alabama)
- Dr. Bruce Lytle (Ohio)

- Dr. Patrick McCarthy (Illinois)
- Dr. Jock McCollough (New Jersey)
- Dr. Tomislav Mihaljevic (Ohio)
- Dr. Craig Miller (California)
- Dr. Mehmet Oz (New York)
- Dr. Gosta Pettersson (Ohio)
- Dr. Eric Roselli (Ohio)
- Dr. William Ryan (Texas)
- Dr. Richard Shemin (California)
- Dr. Vaughn Starnes (California)
- Dr. Paul Stelzer (New York)
- Dr. Lars Svensson (Ohio)
- Dr. Jeffrey Swanson (Oregon)
- Dr. Alfredo Trento (California)
- Dr. Benoit de Varennes (Quebec, Canada)

The second reason I selected Dr. Starnes was based upon his track record specific to the Ross Procedure. Dr. Starnes had performed over two hundred Ross Procedures, while Dr. Trento had performed over one hundred Ross Procedures.

Scheduling The Surgery

I was now ready to schedule my operation. I knew which operation I would have. I knew which surgeon would operate on me.

I nervously called Dr. Starnes' office and spoke with Sherrie, the coordinator. We agreed that on December 21, 2005, I would have open-heart surgery. *That was contingent, however, on how the surgery would be paid for.*

Former Valve Surgery Patient Quote: DeWayne Epley (Georgia)

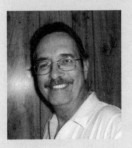

"Don't be afraid to ask questions. No question is un-important as long as it helps you to get ready for things to come. Read as much as you can to become as familiar with circumstances and procedures and options. The better prepared you are... The better your experience will be."

"Did You Travel For Heart Valve Surgery?" Asks Carol

Adam's Heart Valve Surgery Blog Excerpt - Posted September 25, 2009

I just received a great question from Carol about traveling for heart valve surgery. She writes, "I have concerns about choosing a hospital that is highly regarded for valve replacement surgery but out of town. Have any of your readers traveled significant distances for their surgeries? Were there any problems? How did they handle follow-ups? Thanks, Carol"

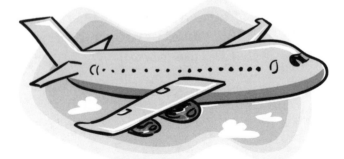

Carol raises a very good point. In fact, her email reminded me of my gut reaction when I was diagnosed with severe aortic stenosis and told I needed surgery.

"Even though I live in California, I'm going to The Cleveland Clinic or The Mayo Clinic!" I thought to myself. "No messing around… I want the best surgeon… That surgeon must be in Ohio or Minnesota."

So you know, that is a very, very, very common thought among many of the patients and caregivers I have spoken with over the years. Interestingly enough, that thought often turns into reality for some patients.

I recently learned that in 2008:

- Over 50% of heart surgery patients at The Cleveland Clinic were not residents of Ohio (e.g. Robin Williams);
- Patients from 89 countries came to The Cleveland Clinic for cardiovascular care; and
- Patients from all 50 states came to The Cleveland Clinic for cardiac surgery.

However, when I took the time to research and evaluate surgeons for the procedure I wanted, I found some heart valve gurus right in my own backyard.

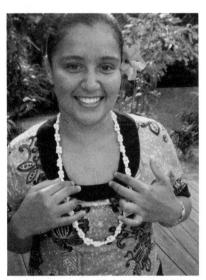

Mary Billings – Traveled From Fiji To Los Angeles For Heart Valve Surgery
(Source: Adam Pick)

I admit… I was lucky. This is often not the case for many, many, many patients out there. As a result, patients must travel - by car, by plane, by train - to have surgery done. In fact, I know patients from Fiji, Trinidad, Somalia, The Philippines and Malaysia that have traveled to the United States for surgery.

The points I am trying to make are two-fold:

- First, each patient case is unique. Please take the time to evaluate your surgical needs. Then, research the surgeons and hospitals that provide the best care for you.

- Second, traveling for heart valve surgery does occur - and, quite frequently. That said, many hospitals have services to make your pre- and post-operative time very manageable.

I hope this helps you better understand traveling for heart valve surgery. Let's see what our community has to say about this.

Keep on tickin!

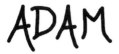

P.S. As you would imagine, several patients posted comments to this blog located at http://www.heart-valve-surgery.com/heart-surgery-blog/2009/09/25/travel-heart-surgery-stenosis/.

- Debbie said, "I traveled from Chicago to North Carolina because I was told that Dr. Randolph Chitwood had done more robotic mitral valve repairs. In total, I was away from home for approximately ten days. That included five days in the hospital. Post surgery, my husband and I stayed at a hotel close to Pitt County Memorial Hospital. I saw the doctors twice before leaving North Carolina. One of the surgeons even came to our hotel on the day we were leaving to make sure that all was okay. Now, I see my own cardiologist at Northwestern Hospital. If you have confidence in a particular doctor, I would not hesitate to travel."

- Darrin said, "I traveled to the Mayo Clinic so that Dr. Rakesh Suri could do my mitral valve repair robotically (minimally invasive). Mayo also publishes stats that indicate more than 50% of their patients travel 500 miles or more for treatment at Mayo. I had no issues with the travel. I am pleased with the results and would do it again."

• Marlane said, "I live in Tucson, Arizona and I traveled by plane to San Francisco to have Dr. Gaudiani perform my aortic valve replacement. I was in the hospital six days. Then, I went to a hotel that was very close to the hospital for three days. I then boarded an airplane and flew home without a problem. You really need to work with the hospital and do all the pre-op work they ask you to do. I had no problems at all."

• Nancy said, "I live about 30 miles south of Boston and my cardiologist is in Plymouth, Massachusetts. When he diagnosed me with severe aortic stenosis, he recommended a surgeon at Brigham and Women's in Boston who turned out to be world famous! My point is... If you have a cardiologist that you can trust, research his recommendations. Traveling any long distance would have been difficult for me right after surgery. I felt every little bump in the road on the way home from Boston and I was in a comfortable limo! But, as Adam says, everyone is different!"

The Costs Of Heart Valve Surgery

In this chapter, you will:
- Learn about the fees associated with heart valve surgery.
- Become aware of the challenges in paying for heart valve surgery.
- Review my case study about heart valve surgery costs.

My number one priority for heart valve surgery focused on finding the right surgeon. I remember thinking, "Money is no object for this procedure. I don't care what it costs. I want to find the best surgeon. I want the best care. I will go anywhere to have this done. I'll worry about the fees afterward."

 A long time ago a friend once said to me, "When you die, the money in your bank account is irrelevant." That might be cliche, but I believe it. That is why I was so adamant about finding the top surgeon.

Still, one of the most curious questions I had about heart valve surgery was, "How much is this operation going to cost me?"

Unfortunately, no one seemed to have a reliable answer to that question. My uncle told me, "A procedure like that will probably cost in the six figures." Another buddy said, "My cousin had some valve work done... I hear it cost two hundred thousand bucks."

I then went to the Internet and searched for an answer. I never really found anything that detailed how much heart valve surgery actually cost the patient.

It was quite frustrating.

Eventually, I found three references to heart valve surgery costs from Columbia University, The National Library of Medicine and East Carolina University. Here is what they said:

- *Columbia University.* Between 1992 and 1997, length of hospital stay decreased from 13.4 to 8.0 days and cost decreased from $37,047 to $21,856. Similarly, between 1992 and 1997 for mitral valve repair, length of stay decreased from 15.6 to 8.1 days and cost decreased from $45,072 to $21,747. The net result over the time period from 1988 to 1997 was an average decline in the cost of operation of $785 a year, adjusted for other factors.

- *National Library of Medicine.* Cost per patient was $14,469 for mitral valve replacement, and $11,606 for mitral valve repair.

- At *East Carolina University*, surgeons say that the hospital receives a fixed fee of $25,000 for the total cost of each heart valve repair regardless of whether robotics are used.

The cost estimates from the medical resources significantly varied from my friend's estimates. My friends were telling me the procedure would cost over $100,000 while the medical journals were telling me the medical fees would be around $25,000.

Your Financial Responsibility Is Unique To You

When you review these estimates, a fundamental question arises, "Why is there such a great variance in the estimated costs of heart valve surgery?"

I had no confident answer to that question when I began this research. However, as I talked to more people and learned about the complex billing systems of hospitals, surgeons, cardiologist and insurance companies I began to understand a critical finding that I will share with you now.

 Your financial responsibility will be unique to your own situation.

What do I mean by that statement? I mean that medical fees are determined by several elements that will determine your own, out-of-pocket costs. There is no one standard fee for any operation. The total fees for heart valve surgery will vary and depend on several factors.

For example, consider the different *health insurance providers* which exist today - Blue Shield, HealthNet, Pacificare, Cigna, Assuarant, Blue Cross. Each medical plan has its own terms-and-conditions with each of the doctors and facilities you will use during your operation and hospital stay.

Taken one step further, consider the different *health care plans* offered by the various insurance companies – health maintenance organization (HMO), preferred provider organization (PPO), point-of-service organization (POS) and out-of-network plans. Each plan has its own terms-and-conditions between you and your insurance company which ultimately defines your financial liability.

Furthermore, there are a number of federal (e.g. Medicare) and state programs (e.g. Medi-Cal) that are designed to cover the special needs of certain demographic groups (e.g. age). For example, Medicare covers over 38 million people in the United States.

Case Study – Heart Valve Surgery Costs
Patient: Adam Pick

To give you some perspective on the costs of heart valve surgery, I just spent thirty minutes looking through all of my medical bills for the past year. It was quite interesting research. Before I give you the financial details, here is my background as it relates to this surgery:

- I was a thirty-three year old male at the time of surgery.
- I held a point-of-service insurance plan with Blue Shield of California which was provided to me by work.
- My cardiologist, my surgeon and my hospital fees were not in the HMO portion of my plan so I was required to pay 20% of my total fees with a maximum out-of-pocket limit of $2,000.

In reviewing my statements, I learned that forty-nine claims were processed through Blue Shield which related to my operation. The total billed amount of those claims was $224,500.

I then reviewed my bank records and credit card statements to determine how much money I spent on fees related to my diagnosis and surgery. My out-of-pocket expenses were about $4,900. (Those fees would have been lower, however, I chose to have some medical testing done outside of my insurance plan coverage.)

12/21/05	USCAN ANESTHESIOLOGY	$4,270.00
12/21/05	USCAN ANESTHESIOLOGY	$4,270.00
12/21/05	USC CARDIOTHORACIC SURGEONS	$1,780.00
12/21/05	USC CARDIOTHORACIC SURGEONS	$8,900.00
12/21/05	USC INTERNAL MEDICINE INC	$1,145.00
12/21/05	USC RADIOLOGY ASSOCS	$30.00
12/21/05-12/25/05	USC UNIVERSITY HOSPITAL	$187,040.89
12/20/05-12/21/05	UNIVERSITY PATH ASSOCS INC	$417.00
12/20/05	UNIVERSITY PATH ASSOCS INC	$67.00
12/20/05	USC RADIOLOGY ASSOCS	$36.00
12/20/05	USC RADIOLOGY ASSOCS	$36.00

Select Adam Pick Medical Expenses
(Source: Blue Shield of California)

As I reviewed my statement, I was amazed to find a claim for $187,040 billed by USC University Hospital. That's a lot of money! However, as I looked further into the details of this claim, I noticed that my insurance company only paid $21,032.17 of the original $187,040 claim. That's a huge difference!

After speaking with a doctor friend of mine, I learned that hospitals and doctors can submit claims for almost any amount to the patient's insurance company. However, insurance providers are only obligated to pay the amount referenced in their contracts with the doctor or hospital.

Claim Detail			
Service Details			**Blue SI**
Date(s) of Service ⑦	**Type of Service/Procedure Number**	**Amount Billed** ⑦	**Amount Allowed** ⑦
12/21/2005 - 12/25/2005	ICU/CCU performed at Hospital inpatient	$9,093.00	$23,017.00
12/21/2005 - 12/25/2005	ICU/CCU performed at Hospital inpatient	$996.00	$0.00
12/21/2005 - 12/25/2005	ICU/CCU performed at Intensive care/coronary care unit	$9,155.00	$0.00
12/21/2005 - 12/25/2005	HOSP MISC performed at Hospital inpatient	$134,913.89	$0.00
12/21/2005 - 12/25/2005	MEDICAL EQUIP performed at Hospital inpatient	$32,533.00	$0.00
12/21/2005 - 12/25/2005	MEDICAL EQUIP performed at Hospital inpatient	$350.00	$0.00
	Claim Totals:	$187,040.89	$23,017.00

Details of $187,040 Bill From USC University Hospital
(Source: Blue Shield of California)

So, after reviewing my records and the records of my healthcare provider, it appears that the cost of my surgery was really only about $33,000, although the billed amount for the surgery was approximately $224,500. And, as for me, I paid about $4,900 or 14% of the real costs.

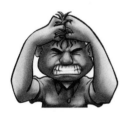

Be Prepared to Get Frustrated With Insurance Companies!

As you interact with your insurance provider, your doctors and the hospital about surgery costs, you may get frustrated. Insurance agents may not have immediate answers to your questions. Or, you may be put on hold for long periods of time. And, you may get conflicting information.

I remember a phone call to my insurance company in which I was on hold for ninety minutes only to be told that I was calling the wrong phone number.

Are you ready for the worst experience? On the day of my surgery, I was in the pre-operating room getting ready for surgery. The anesthesiologist had already given me a few pills to help calm me down. Minutes before I was wheeled into the operating room, a hospital administrator asked me for my credit card.

I had to sign a credit card slip just a few minutes before surgery!

My point... Be prepared for a little frustration.

Your Support Group

In this chapter, you will:
- Learn the importance of friends and family specific to your heart valve surgery.
- The need to effectively share information with your support group.
- Get inspired by our *second* heart valve surgery success story.

Now, for the really, really, really, really important stuff! This may be the most important chapter of the book. I encourage you to read this section with great attention and curiosity.

Interestingly enough, this chapter has very little to do with you. That's right. It's the first-and-only chapter in *The Patient's Guide To Heart Valve Surgery* that will actually focus on anything but you.

Instead, it focuses on the people around you – your support group.

Let me explain...

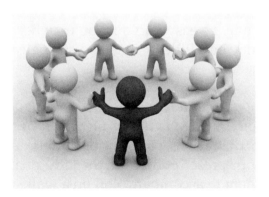

Communicating Your Needs

While you are personally experiencing the reality of heart valve surgery, the people around you - your friends, your family, your coworkers - will also experience this process with you. You may not know it yet, but there is a great, growing awareness to your condition.

Personally, I was amazed and very pleased to see how my friends, family and coworkers reacted to the news that I would be having heart surgery. There was a rally of support that really picked me up through this trying time. As you might imagine, I really appreciated the 'cheerleading' that came from my support group.

Leading up to the surgery, however, all of that support became overwhelming. It seemed as if everyone I knew had an opinion about my surgeon or the procedure I selected.

Deep down, I knew that everyone was trying to help and comfort me but I remember several conversations where I had to ask members of my support group to stop providing me with new information, new website links and new referrals.

 One of the most important lessons I learned during my heart valve surgery experience was to communicate with my support group.

During the pre-operation, operation and post-operation phases, it is critical that you share what is on your mind with your friends, family and co-workers.

This type of communication may be easy for you. You may be a Dr. Phil or Oprah disciple. Alternatively, you may be a little like me and struggle when it comes to sharing your thoughts and needs.

Regardless of your skills, *you will need to communicate with your support group to ensure they know what you need and want during this process.* At times, you may need to talk about your frustrations, concerns or doubts. At other times, you may need them to pick-up your prescription from the local pharmacy. And, at other times, you may want them to accompany you on a walk.

While your need to communicate will elevate during your recovery, it does not hurt to get started now. Remember, your support group is there to 'support' you.

Managing Expectations

Personally, I found that managing expectations was critical for my friends and family. Most people are not familiar with the realities of heart valve surgery. Accordingly, most people tend to fear what they do not know about.

You may want to sit down with your friends and family and explain your medical condition and how you are going to fix it. Like you, they are bound to have questions.

 It might help your support group if you openly discuss the details of heart valve surgery with them. Or, you may want to give them a copy of this book, so they can learn more about the surgery on their own time.

In addition to talking with my support group, I found email to be a very effective tool for communicating and managing expectations. For example, a few days before my surgery, I wrote an email to my support group. I wanted each and every person to know what was happening the day of the surgery and the weeks following.

Here is a copy of that email:

From: Adam Pick
Date: Mon, 19 Dec 2005
Subject: Update

Family and Friends,

Just thought I would give you a quick update and make sure you are aware of what's happening over the next few weeks.

* On Wednesday, Robyn will be taking me to USC. We will arrive at 7am for the 9am operation. The procedure is expected to last 3-4 hours.

* It is expected that I will be in the ICU for the first 24 hours following the procedure. Thereafter, I will be moved to a room that may or may not be private. According to Dr. Starnes office, there is a very, very high probability I will have a private room for my entire stay. I am expected

to be in the hospital for 5-7 days.

* As for the recovery, after I leave the hospital, I have chosen to stay in Redondo Beach. While Monie and Robert have been super, ultra loving with their offer to recover in Newport, I really would like to simply be home. I will be talking to each of you in the next 24 hours to discuss the ways in which you can support me during this time (2-3 weeks). Please see attached.

* So you know, the address of the hospital is 1500 San Pablo St., Los Angeles, CA 90033 (map attached), (323) 442-8500. The phone number for Dr. Starnes office is (323) 442-5849

* Thanks again for all of your love and help!!!

Love... Ad

Heart Valve Journals! Helping You Stay Connected!

As you might agree, the email referenced above is not enough information to keep your support group "updated" or "in the loop" as you transition from diagnosis to surgery into recovery.

For that reason, I developed a very special, online tool known as Heart Valve Journals. This free program was designed to stimulate ongoing communication and interaction among you and your caregivers.

Once you create a Heart Valve Journal, you can:

- Write your own journals (blogs) to keep everybody informed on your health status and condition.
- Upload pictures so friends and family can see and learn about your experience.
- Interact with your support group through a special Internet feature called the Guestbook.

Also, Heart Valve Journals enables your caregivers to subscribe to your journal by email and RSS feed. That way, every time you update your Heart Valve Journal, your friends and family will know about it!

Finally, this online community gives you a rare opportunity to meet and learn from other patients all over the world.

To set up your free journal, please go to **www.HeartValveJournals.com**.

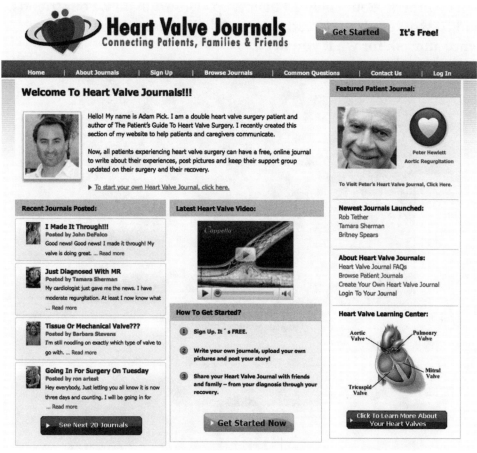

(www.HeartValveJournals.com)

A Little Bit Of Dependence Doesn't Hurt

In closing this section, I strongly encourage you to consider that your support group will become a critical factor in your recovery. As you transition from the intensive care unit, to your hospital bed, back to your home, the people around you will play an incredibly important role in your physical and mental well-being.

Take the appropriate time before your surgery to make sure that you are all on the same page. The invasive nature of this surgery will temporarily make you a little dependent on others. You will need their help. Unfortunately, your friends, family and co-workers can not read your mind. **Embrace this temporary dependence and ask for what you need.**

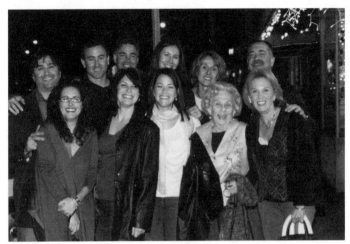

My Support Group
(Source: Monica Cohen)

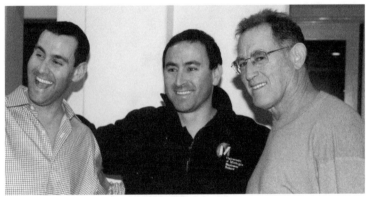

My Brother (Doug), Me, My Dad (Jerry)
(Source: Monica Cohen)

Heart Valve Surgery Success Story:
David Watkins, The Ironman Legacy
(Source: Adult Congenital Heart Association, David Watkins)

In 2002, after training for triathlon competition (a threepart endurance event involving swimming, cycling, and running), David's heartbeat raced from 150 beats per minute to 170, then past 200.

"By then all I could do was grab the shoulders of my wife and dad before I went down," said David. With no history of heart problems, this was David's first indication that something was terribly wrong.

David was initially diagnosed with a bicuspid aortic valve (he had two leaflets instead of three). Since his valve seemed to be functioning just fine, David continued to train for triathlons and adventure races. The arrythmias continued, too.

After two frustrating years of visits with multiple cardiologists and incorrect diagnoses, Dr. Salerno, at University of Washington Medical Center, diagnosed David with a dilated ascending aorta, hypertension, and atrial fibrillation. During a subsequent cardiac check-up, David was also diagnosed with an aneurysm of the ascending aorta—a ballooning of the blood's major route from the heart to the rest of his body.

Dr. Salerno advised David that without surgery, he was at significant risk for sudden death. His aorta could rupture at any time. On May 20, 2005, the surgery that was scheduled to take five hours to replace the aortic root, turned into ten. David's ballooning aortic valve was worse than expected. Rather than replacing just the root, the aortic valve also had to be replaced.

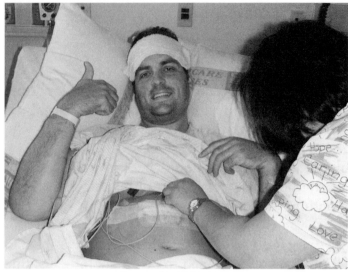

(Source: David Watkins)

Following surgery, David was taken to the intensive care unit where his wife, Kerri, joined him. That is when the second phase of David's heart triathlon began. David's fast heart rate, this time in another heart chamber, returned in the form of ventricular fibrillation. His heart stopped for five minutes.

Before wheeling him back into surgery, Kerri was asked if she had any last words for David. She simply said, "Fight and be strong." He needed to do just that as he underwent a successful five-hour coronary artery by-pass surgery.

The event was not yet over. After recovering at home for one week, David ate some Chinese take-out food. He bloated up and his heartbeat jumped to 160. Doctors later determined the probable cause was an allergic reaction to shellfish — the allergy had been transmitted to David through one of his many blood transfusions. But no one knew that at the time.

Fearing the worst, David was raced back to the hospital where doctors shocked him for atrial flutter. After his heart returned to a normal rhythm and he was stabilized for another week, David was sent home. Two days later, on Father's Day, David had a slight stroke, which caused a temporary loss of vision in his left eye and feeling on the left side of his face.

Upon returning home, David felt that his body was ready for the healing process to begin. He told his family that he was going to start training for the Ironman Triathlon, just 13 months away.

"I had always dreamt of doing an Ironman triathlon," says David. "But I never had the discipline or vision to complete it. Most importantly, right before surgery, I made a promise to myself that if I survived, I would begin leaving a legacy to my daughters, Maya and Madeline (then ages 7 and 4). That legacy was a 'life lesson.' I wanted them to always remember 'no matter what obstacles life throws at you, no matter what odds are stacked against you, if you believe in yourself, you can and will accomplish amazing things.' There was no better way of teaching them this message than by example."

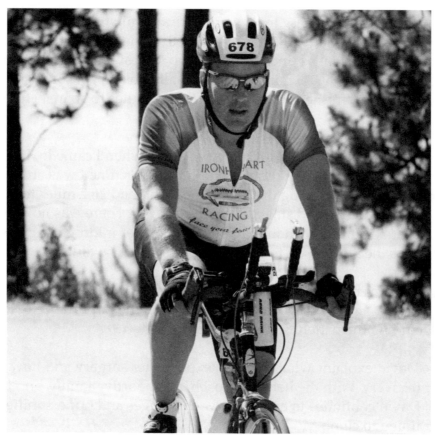

(Source: David Watkins)

While other competitors may have begun their training by cycling or running, David's began "by getting from the couch to the bathroom on my own. Then, it was from the couch to the kitchen. Soon, I was out the door to the end of the driveway. Next, I made it to the mailbox, and soon after that, the end of the block."

Six months later, David completed the 2005 Seattle Half-Marathon, a 13.1 mile run. Seven months after that, David stood at the Ironman Triathlon starting line. Competition began with swimming, the event David trained hardest for. He came out 45 minutes ahead of his expected pace. But this was followed by his toughest event in the Ironman Triathlon—bicycling. While on this 112 mile endurance race, David's heart rate monitor and bike computer malfunctioned.

David recalls it this way: "These tools were critical to my training, and now I was without them. To make matters worse, at mile 60, my left cleat broke and I had to pedal approximately 30 miles (including the two largest hills) with only my right foot clipped into my pedal. At mile 90, I was finally able to get some assistance and fix my left cleat. I finished the bike with four minutes to spare before the cutoff.

"It took two people to physically lift me off my bike when I came in. I could barely run, let alone stand erect. It also didn't help that by this time I was able to hear plenty of racers already crossing the finish line. I still had 26.2 miles to run. Kerri snuck out onto the course and stayed with me as I ran. There was no way I would have been able to continue without her. Some time after midnight, I crossed the finish line. I was the last person to make it." But make it he did.

Today, David shares his story and competitive spirit with other patients and surgeons. His message to surgeons is this: "I explain the importance of knowing and understanding the patient's goals after surgery."

To patients, David explains what they can expect after surgery and how best to prepare for recovery. With the help of a coach, a supportive family, and his team of physicians, David continues to explore new challenges and opportunities. He is currently training to climb Mt. Rainier in 2008.

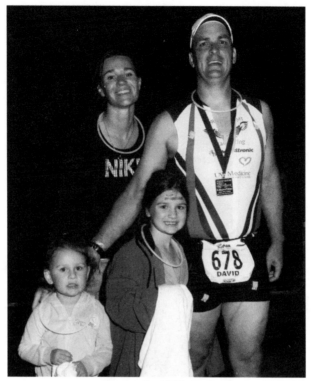

(Source: David Watkins)

PART III
THE HEART VALVE
OPERATION

Preparing For Surgery

In this chapter, you will:
- Learn about the final medical tests and labs before admission.
- Read about some helpful items to bring with you to the hospital.
- Review select survey results regarding the *hospital experience*.

We have covered a lot of information in this book. We have dispelled the fears of heart valve surgery. We have examined the anatomy of the heart and its valves. We have learned the surgical procedures to fix heart valve disorders. We addressed how to find the right surgeon. We have talked about the cost of heart valve surgery. And, we have discussed the importance of your support group.

Part III of *The Patient's Guide To Heart Valve Surgery* focuses specifically on your time in the hospital. I will cover what occurs for the patient once he or she enters the hospital, undergoes surgery and then proceeds through the beginning stages of recovery. For your reference, a heart valve surgery patient typically stays in the hospital for four to seven days.

To start, this chapter will discuss the final steps leading up to your admission in the hospital. So you know, there really is not much to do prior to your admission. However, there are some things you should know that might make your hospital stay a little more comfortable.

Let's start with what you need to do leading up to your surgery!!!

Lab Work And Tests Prior To Surgery

Leading up to your surgery, you may be asked to visit the hospital to have a series of tests performed. These tests may include:

- **Blood tests** – Your blood will be screened for disease and tested for blood type.

- **Electrocardiogram** – An electrocardiogram records the electrical activity of the heart over time. It provides cardiac rhythm analysis and plays a key role in the screening and diagnosis of cardiovascular disease.

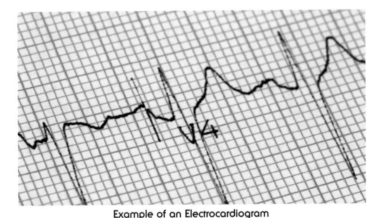

Example of an Electrocardiogram

- **Angiogram** – An angiogram is an imaging test that uses x-rays to view your body's blood vessels. Physicians often use this test to study narrow, blocked, enlarged, or malformed arteries in many parts of your body, including your brain, heart, abdomen, and legs. When the arteries are studied, the test is also called an arteriogram. If the veins are studied, it is called a venogram.

- **Urine analysis** – As well as removing waste from the body, urine can be examined to determine many medical conditions concerning the bladder, kidneys, and even metabolic functions of the body.

Banking Your Blood?

As you are learning, patients are faced with many, many, many questions prior to heart surgery. One additional question is specific to *potential* blood loss during the operation. That said, you may hear this question in the days or weeks before surgery, *"Would you like to donate blood or use blood from the hospital blood bank?"*

Personally, I did not donate my own blood prior to surgery. However, I just read an interesting article at the *Mercury News* which reveals that heart surgery patients treated with donated blood older than two weeks were more likely to die or suffer problems than those treated with fresher blood.

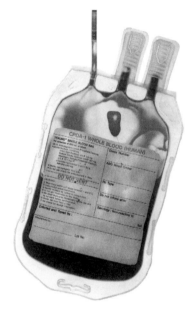

These findings are even more problematic when you consider that blood supplies are chronically low.

"If the shelf life was reduced from 42 to 14 days, we just wouldn't have enough blood around," said Dr. Ross Herron, medical director of the American Red Cross Bay Area, which sends blood to hospitals throughout the East Bay and South Bay. "We need to have that shelf life to move blood around."

As noted above, I did not donate my own blood prior to heart valve surgery.

(Luckily, Dr. Starnes did not need to perform a transfusion during my surgery.) However, given these findings, I would probably change that approach if I needed heart surgery again.

Consent For Surgery

Upon completion of your tests and lab work, you may also be required to sign a legal document that illustrates your consent to have surgery. Prior to signing the consent, a member of your medical team (surgeon, resident, intern) will take about thirty minutes to review the surgical process and answer any final questions you may have.

During this discussion, the doctor will also review the medical risks associated with heart valve surgery. This can be very challenging to hear and digest. Personally, I was quite shocked when my doctor reviewed the potential problems (e.g. stroke) of heart valve surgery.

However, I had complete faith in my surgeon and his medical team. I had taken the proper steps to find the right surgeon for me. Also, by this time, my fears about heart valve surgery were dispelled (see Chapter One), so I grabbed the pen and signed the form.

That's it. I was now ready to be admitted for surgery the next morning at seven o'clock.

What To Bring To The Hospital?

Now that you are officially ready for surgery, it's time to stop and consider that you will be away from home for several days. That said, you may want to think about what might make your stay in the hospital more comfortable.

Here are a couple things that I brought with me:

- Pillow
- Robe
- Toothbrush and toothpaste
- Slippers

- Pajamas
- Loose fitting clothes (sweat pants, sweat shirt)
- Book / journal
- Hearos ear plugs
- Apple iPod
- Mobile phone
- Camera

As for clothes, you will most likely be in a gown for most of your time in the hospital. Therefore, you do not need to bring but one change of clothes with you to the hospital. I left the hospital in my pajamas and my robe.

In addition to the physical items you bring to the hospital, I also believe that patients should bring some invisible items as well. Here are my *"Top 5 Invisible Things To Bring To The Hospital":*

1. **Courage** – Even though statistics suggest your surgical result will be good, that might not stop the fear, uncertainty and doubt that impacts most patients. Courage became one of my best friends in the hospital.

2. **Trust** - Patients should bring A LOT of trust with them to the hospital. Trust in the hospital. Trust in their support group. And, most importantly, trust in their surgeon. If you don't have trust, DO NOT go to the hospital! Step back from this process and conduct more diligence on your diagnosis, your procedure and your surgeon.

3. **Healthy Thoughts** – You are what you think about. That said, think healthy thoughts and you will become healthy.

4. **Patience** - Once surgery is complete, patients immediately enter the recovery process. However, as you will soon read, recovering from heart surgery can be challenging. Within the first 24 hours after surgery, I realized how critical the cliche "Patience is a virtue" is for heart surgery patients. Patients need to be patient!

5. **Love** - Bring A LOT of love to the hospital. As the heart is the international symbol of love, it really helped me to share love with my wife, my friends,

my family, my medical team, and most importantly… my newly stitched heart.

Survey Results - The Hospital Experience

Now that you are prepared to enter the hospital, it makes sense to prepare you for the hospital experience. Many patients have conflicting thoughts, feelings and emotions as they enter the hospital.

Some patients are excited.

Some patients are scared.

Some patients are nervous.

So you know, those feelings are all normal and rational.

Mostly, patients experience a dominant feeling of uncertainty. I remember being concerned about the uncertainty of the surgery. I also remember being concerned about the uncertainty of life in the hospital after the surgery.

Well… I can tell you now, fifteen months after surgery, living in a hospital for a few days was not that bad. The doctors, nurses and therapists at USC Medical Center did an excellent job at making my family and I very comfortable during those five days I spent in the hospital.

Still, I was curious to know if my experience was similar to other patients. So, I recently surveyed several patients about their experience in their respective hospitals.

The results were quite interesting.

First, I wanted to know how long heart valve surgery patients were in the hospital following surgery. As you can see below, the average patient spent five days in the hospital.

Those patients, which spent ten or more days in the hospital, typically experienced some form of post-operative complication which required them to receive additional care and a longer hospital stay.

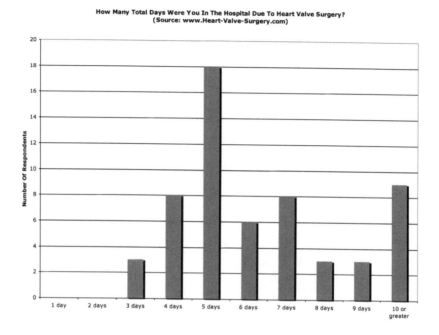

How Many Total Days Were You In The Hospital Due To Heart Valve Surgery?
(Source: www.Heart-Valve-Surgery.com)

Then, I asked the survey respondents about their feelings toward their hospital experience. I asked each of them to complete the following sentence, "My hospital experience was _____."

I provided the patients with five potential answers: *excellent, good, fair, difficult and terrible.*

As you can see, the majority of patients were quite happy with their experience in the hospital.

According to our survey, most heart valve surgery patients described their hospital experience as *excellent* (46%) or *good* (34%). That's pretty amazing! Eighty percent of respondents had positive things to say about their time in the hospital following heart valve surgery.

Patients Felt Their Experience In The Hospital Was _____.
(Source: www.Heart-Valve-Surgery.com)

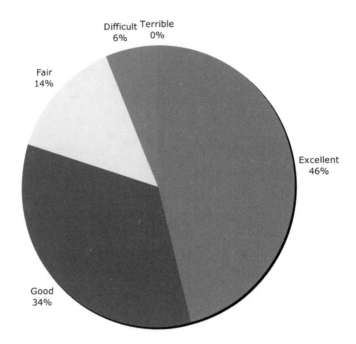

Difficult Terrible
6% 0%

Fair
14%

Excellent
46%

Good
34%

During the survey and research process, I even learned that some patients and caregivers were incredibly fond of their hospitals. I have listed below, for your review, a number of the cardiac surgery centers that received the most praise from the patients and caregivers surveyed:

- Barnes-Jewish Hospital / Washington University (Missouri)
- Brigham and Women's Hospital (Massachusetts)
- Cedars-Sinai Medical Center (California)
- The Cleveland Clinic (Ohio)
- Dallas Presbyterian Hospital (Texas)
- Duke University Medical Center (North Carolina)
- Emory University Hospital (Georgia)
- Good Samaritan Hospital (California)
- Jefferson Regional Medical Center (Pennsylvania)

- Johns Hopkins Hospital (Maryland)
- Massachusetts General Hospital (Massachusetts)
- Mayo Clinic (Minnesota)
- Mount Sinai Medical Center (New York)
- New York Presbyterian University Hospital (New York)
- Northwestern Memorial Hospital (Illinois)
- Ochsner Foundation Hospital (Louisiana)
- St. Peter's Hospital (Washington)
- Texas Heart Institute (Texas)
- Toronto General Hospital (Canada)
- USC Medical Center (California)
- Washoe Medical Center (Nevada)
- West Florida Hospital (Florida)

The data provided above should reassure you that your time in the hospital will most likely be well managed and comfortable. If you look back at the chart above, you will notice that not one patient deemed their hospital experience as *terrible*.

The Night Before Surgery...

I was nervous the night before surgery. To ease my anxiety, I called several members of my support group to tell them how much I loved and cared for them. It was a very special, emotional evening. I cried a lot. They cried a lot.

I will never forget the phone call with my brother, Doug. While talking about the surgery, a power greater than myself arose from within and spoke to Doug. While I was in tears, that powerful force said, "Tomorrow will be a great day!"

Doug confirmed, "Yes. Tomorrow, you will start the next chapter of your life."

To help me sleep, my doctor gave me a Xanax. The pill worked like a charm. I slept like a baby and woke up the next morning ready for my aortic and pulmonary valve replacement surgery.

"Did You Exercise Before Heart Valve Surgery?" Asks Leticia

Adam's Heart Valve Surgery Blog Excerpt – Posted On August 10, 2009

I just received a great question from Leticia about exercise prior to heart valve surgery.

Leticia writes, "Hi Adam, I have been diagnosed with a bicuspid aortic heart valve. I have no symptoms or shortness of breath. My cardiologist hopes I can go for another 10 years without surgery. I'm concerned about my hobbies, which are aerobics and I teach ballet. I love my exercise and my doctor states that I don't have to change my lifestyle unless I'm feeling symptoms. I've just read stories about athletic people having to reduce activity until after surgery. I don't want to pass out one day and seriously injure or kill myself. Do you have any other info on exercise and bi-cuspid aortic heart valve? Thank you, Leticia"

As Leticia alludes, valvular disorders can negatively impact heart function during exercise for patients prior to heart valve surgery.

In fact, I just posted a patient story about Randy, from Wisconsin, who fainted while bike riding due to a bicuspid aortic valve. (Thankfully, everything worked out okay for Randy.)

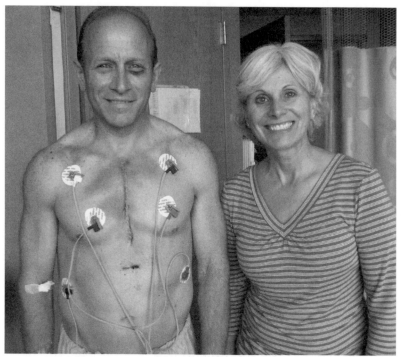

Randy Heimerl – Heart Valve Surgery Patient – With Cheryl, His Wife
(Source: Randy Heimerl)

At the same time, other patients - under medical supervision - engage in exercise to enhance their physical condition prior to heart valve surgery. For example, Sylvia Woolworth lost 35 pounds leading up to her heart valve replacement.

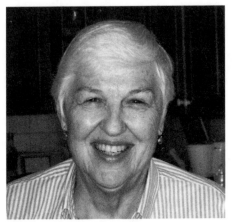

Sylvia Woolworth – Heart Valve Surgery Patient
(Source: Sylvia Woolworth)

As for me, my cardiologist restricted all exercise when it was determined that I needed an aortic valve replacement.

I do not know the specific details of Leticia's valve disease progression (e.g. mild, moderate, or severe). That said, I would suggest that Leticia contact her cardiologist to better understand the severity of the disorder and its impact upon her exercise routine, if any.

One last note… **I would also suggest to Leticia that symptom manifestation may not be the best, definitive indicator for timing heart valve surgery.** So you know, I was asymptomatic but my heart was already enlarged. That said, I think all patients should be actively monitored on a yearly basis following initial diagnosis.

I hope that helps explain a little more about exercise before heart surgery!

Keep on tickin!

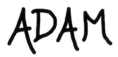

chapter

10

The Morning Of The Operation

In this chapter, you will:
- Learn about the hospital admission process.
- Better understand what happens in the pre-operating and operating rooms.
- Read about the intensive care unit.

I have to admit, when I woke up on the day of my surgery, I was excited. After two months of waiting, it was finally time. Maybe I was tired of the anxiety? Maybe I was ready to get my heart fixed? Or, maybe I just wanted it to be over?

Regardless, I was in a great mood as Robyn drove me across Los Angeles to the USC Medical Center. Considering it was the winter solstice (the shortest day of the year), the sky was dark as we sped across the 405, the 105, and the 110 freeways at six o'clock in the morning.

When the elevator doors opened on the fifth floor of the hospital, there was my support group waiting. I instantly felt more relaxed knowing that my family was there. My mom, my dad, my dad's girlfriend, my sister, my brother and my aunt all gathered around me as we exchanged a group hug.

After exchanging many *"I love yous"* with my family, I was ready.

I approached the reception area and knocked on the frosted window to check in.

There was no answer.

I knocked again.

Still, no answer.

Immediately I thought, "Oh well, they're closed. I'll come back another day."

Then, three seconds later, the window slid open. I realized they were, in fact, open for business.

I gave the nurse my name and told her I was scheduled for a nine o'clock surgery. She looked at me and said, "Hi Adam. We are running a little behind this morning. Just take a seat and we'll call you when we are ready."

After forty-five minutes of anxious waiting, I finally heard my name called. A female nurse appeared by the door and said, "Adam... We're ready for you in the *pre-operating* room."

I gave my family a final set of hugs, took a very deep breath and followed the nurse.

The Pre-Operating Room

As I passed through the double-doors and entered the pre-operating area, I saw a series of gurneys that were segmented by faded green, medical drapes. It must have been a busy day for heart surgeries because each gurney was filled with a body.

My fellow patients ranged in age from twenty-five to seventy. We held a common bond that morning. We wanted to live. We wanted to be fixed.

My nurse then pointed to the only open gurney in the hall. I entered. She closed the drapes around me.

After taking my blood pressure and my temperature, she listened to my heart and lungs.

"Okay," she said.

I know she told me her name but I have no recollection of anything about that nurse.

"There's a gown," she said as she pointed to the gown and cap that were meticulously folded so neatly in the corner of the area, "You can take off your clothes and get in it. And I... I will be back in a few minutes."

The pre-op area was cold. I decided to take everything off but my sox. I then put on the gown and laid down on the gurney. After ten minutes of waiting, Robyn and my brother, Doug, arrived. It was great having them there with me in my little area.

It was now about nine o'clock in the morning. My surgery was *really* delayed.

I remember thinking, "Come on already. Let's get this going!" Then, moments later, I realized where I was and what could be forcing the delay in my surgery start time.

Maybe the patient in front of me is having severe complications? Maybe Dr. Starnes is in the middle of a heart transplant and something is wrong?

Quickly, I let go of my selfish need to be on time.

A Quick Rotation Of People Dressed In White

No sooner had I relinquished my need to be punctual, that the activity specific to my case went from first to fifth gear. At about nine thirty, a nurse dressed in white appeared, and informed me that it was time to get my *drip* going. Compared with other routes of administration, the intravenous drip is the fastest way to deliver fluids and medications throughout the body. Within seconds, she successfully pierced my vein and disappeared.

My dad, Jerry, then appeared.

Considering that my dad had spent most of his career in an operating room, I waited for him to provide me with some wonderful advice that would explain everything that was happening in that moment.

No such luck. Instead, he offered a rather calm, "Don't worry. It's all going fine. Delays are typical in hospitals."

A few minutes later a very nice nurse arrived at the front of my gurney. She too was dressed in white. She quickly pulled up my chart, saw my name, looked at my dad and said, "Hi Dr. Pick. Wow. It's been awhile." The two of them played catch-up having worked together years ago at a different hospital.

I have no idea what this nurse did while she stood at the foot of my bed. But, she took a good amount of time to do it. She methodically reviewed my chart, made some notes, let out a few "Ah-has" and then left. I don't recall if I ever said one word to her.

The "Full Monty" Body Shave

About ten minutes passed when a male nurse arrived with a power cord in his left hand and an electric shaver in his right hand.

"Wrong room," I thought to myself, "I'm having heart surgery, not brain surgery."

"Mr. Pick?" he questioned as he looked in my direction.

"Yes," I said.

"Hi. My name is Blank," he said with a Latino accent, "I am going to be shaving you for the operation."

"Oh sure," I thought to myself, "He's going to be shaving the hair off my chest. That makes perfect sense!"

I was perfectly wrong. After thirty minutes, I was hairless from the top of my neck to the bottom of my toes. I had just had my first, and hopefully last, body shave.

The Anesthesiologist Takes Over

Five minutes after my shave was completed, the shift began.

It was now time for surgery.

One by one, the nurses stopped appearing.

From here on out, each interaction was with a doctor.

None of them wore white. They all wore blue.

The first doctor to stand by my gurney was Dr. Chu. If I remember right, Dr. Chu was the resident anesthesiologist, probably in his late-twenties.

Dr. Chu was meant to be a doctor. He had a great and comfortable way about him. Dr. Chu told me that we were about thirty minutes away from entering the operating room.

Then, Dr. Haddy, the head anesthesiologist we requested, arrived. He too had a great way about him. He was everything you expect in a doctor. He radiated kindness, competence and caring.

Or, perhaps, I was so nervous that I was projecting all my hopes and dreams for a successful operation onto whomever walked into my draped pre-op area.

Soon after Dr. Haddy reviewed my chart, my dad magically appeared.

After shaking hands, my father questioned Dr. Haddy, "Do you mind if we talk outside for a few minutes?" The two anesthesiologists exited my pre-op area.

Dr. Chu did not hesitate to prepare me for surgery. Shortly after my dad and Dr. Haddy exited the room, Dr. Chu said, "Okay Adam.... We're ready to get this going. I'm going to administer a slight anesthetic to *relax* you."

He squeezed down on a syringe.

I foolishly warned Dr. Chu that I was not going down easy. My insomnia had prepared me for this moment. Dr. Chu smiled and said, "Well, maybe Adam. But, these drugs are pretty strong. Let's just see what happens."

My Gurney, The Surfboard, Takes Me Into Surgery

At first, I felt nothing from the movement of drugs throughout my body.

Dr. Chu told me to relax and that I would see him in the operating room in just a few minutes. Like all of the people who had come before me that morning, Dr. Chu disappeared quickly from the pre-op area.

Still, I felt nothing from the drugs.

"Perhaps, it was just a light anesthetic," I thought to myself, "Dr. Chu must be saving the powerful drugs for the operating room."

Then, out of nowhere, I felt something.

I looked down, over at my right hand.

It was being held in my Aunt Sylvia's hands.

Now, for those of you who don't know my Aunt Syl, I feel somewhat bad for you. She is timeless. She is wise. She is grace. She is one-of-a-kind. And, as a psychologist, she is trained for moments like this.

As my eyelids began to get heavy, Sylvia asked me to picture myself in a peaceful setting. She then tip-toed into the question, "So, where are you Adam?"

I slowly spoke to Sylvia about my peaceful setting. It was the Pacific Ocean.

It was summer time. The sky was clear. The sun was warm. The water was refreshing. I was on my surfboard admiring the beauty of the day. There was a soft breeze floating across my skin.

Dolphins were swimming all around me.

A friendly four-foot wave was approaching me. The wave was breaking right. I began paddling to the wave.

In reality, my gurney was now gliding out of the pre-operating room just as my surfboard was gliding across the ocean's blue waters in my imagination.

It was approximately eleven-thirty in the morning when I entered the operating room.

Samantha Asks, "Will My Mom's Heart Stop During Valve Surgery?"

Adam's Heart Valve Surgery Blog Excerpt - Posted August 18, 2008

In a recent email to me, Samantha writes, "Hi Adam - I'm freaking out right now. My mother was just told that she will need open heart surgery to replace her mitral valve. I am on 'information overload' as I'm surfing the Internet like crazy. I'm trying to better understand the surgical process. Is it true that the heart is stopped during a valve replacement operation? If so, how do they stop the heart?"

Thanks for writing Samantha. I had this exact question as I was getting ready for my aortic valve replacement surgery.

The answer to your first question is "Yes, most likely, your mother's heart will be stopped during her mitral valve replacement." However, you should know that there are certain procedures in which the heart does not necessarily have to stop beating.

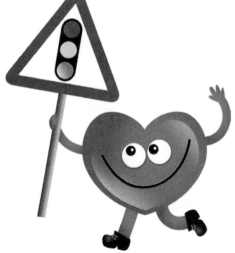

As for your second question, "How will the surgeon stop your mother's heart?", a very unique cooling process will be used to stop your mom's heart. According to the Texas Heart Institute, cooling techniques let surgeons stop the heart for long periods of time without damaging the heart tissue. So you know, cool temperatures avoid damage to the heart tissue by reducing the heart's need for oxygen. The heart may be cooled in two ways:

- Blood is cooled as it passes through the heart-lung machine. In turn, this cooled blood lowers body temperature when it reaches all of the body parts.
- Cold salt-water (saline) is poured over the heart.

After cooling, the heart slows and stops. Injecting a special potassium solution into the heart can speed up this process and stop the heart completely. The heart is then usually safe from tissue injury for 2 to 4 hours.

I would imagine your next question would be, "How the heck do they restart my mom's heart again?" Well, to restart your mother's heart, the surgeon will use a defibrillator.

I'll never forget my reaction when Doctor Starnes explained to me the procedure for cooling, stopping and restarting my heart.

"So let me get this straight," I emphatically questioned the gray-haired guru, "You're going to stop my heart, cool it, fix it and then restart it using an electric shock?"

Doctor Starnes paused, looked calmly into my eyes and then replied with a simple, unemotional one-word response, "Yes."

"Ohhhhhhhhh-kaaaaaay," I slowly muttered in a humble daze as I pondered the magic of modern medicine.

I hope the above information helps you better understand how the heart is stopped and restarted during heart valve surgery.

Keep on tickin!

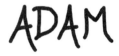

11

Waking Up In The Intensive Care Unit

....

In this chapter, you will:
- · Learn what will happen as you wake up from surgery.
- · Read about my experience in the intensive care unit.

....

I would exit the operating room at three-thirty in the afternoon. The surgery was four hours long. During my research, I have learned that most heart valve operations last between four and six hours.

So you know, I remember nothing of the event.

In-And-Out Of Sleep

The general anesthetic would keep me asleep for another two hours. At about five-thirty in the afternoon, my eyelids separated and, once again, light stimulated my pupils. I was awake.

Seconds after I opened my eyes, I fell back to sleep.

Sometime later, my eyelids would split again. This time, however, I was conscious. I was able to mentally center my attention.

My first cognitive process centered on the image of my father standing before me. He was on the left side of my bed, standing tall, not more than a foot away.

What I then experienced was beautiful.

I saw my father smiling from ear to ear. Even though his hands were in his pockets, there was joy and love radiating from his heart to mine.

I knew the operation went well. He was happy. I was relieved.

I wanted to talk with him. I wanted to know what had happened. I wanted the details.

However, a vent tube prevented that communication. This foreign structure rendered my vocal capability useless. While it was quite uncomfortable, I remained calm and chose to enjoy the silence.

Then, I noticed Robyn behind my father.

I fell back to sleep.

The next time I awoke, my brother Doug was before me. He was holding a sign that said, "You Got Ross, Your Second Birthday, 12/21/05." There were a few smiley faces on the paper as well.

Even though my ability to talk was still constrained, my arms were now free. I lifted my hand and gave him the *thumbs-up* signal. We enjoyed the silence. I did my best to smile even though the vent tube made that difficult.

Again, I noticed Robyn standing a few feet behind Doug.

The Beeps, The Blips, The Bonks, The Gurgling

As I laid quiet in the intensive care unit, I started to notice an amazing assortment of unique sounds dancing across my eardrums. It seemed as if the intensive care unit had its own, continuous symphony of beeps, blips, and bonks sounding in no specific order, with no specific rhythm.

There was also a very deep gurgling noise that continued almost like a bass drum in the background. In addition to the gurgling, there was a swooshing and bubbling component to it.

As the symphony continued, I fell back to sleep.

The Vent Tube And The Water

The next time I awoke I immediately noticed the vent tube. While I knew this medical device was critical to my well-being, it was growing more and more uncomfortable as it irritated my lips, my tongue and my very dry throat.

I did my best to relax and forget its presence.

This time my mom, Donna, was in the room. While I do not remember seeing her, I do remember hearing her voice and her occasional, nervous laugh.

I signaled to my mouth. My mouth was dry and chapped. Moments later, my mouth was being dabbed with a moist, sponge-like tool which released six wonderful water drops onto my tongue. I wanted more. But, the ICU nurse, Blythe, forbid it.

Something was about to happen.

"It's time to take it out," I remember hearing in the background. The statement echoed in my head, as my chemical-induced body, processed the information. I then heard and felt a bustle around me.

I remember hearing Blythe say, "Adam, we are going to take the tube out now."

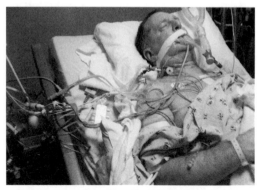

Patient In Intensive Care Unit With Ventilator Tube Inserted
(Photo of Charles Alexander, Courtesy of Jane Chafin)

There was no countdown. There was no warning. In the following moment, the snake-like coil slithered up my chest, through my throat and out my mouth.

I do not remember the first words formed by my liberated voice.

The Catheter Confuses Me

As I continued to regain consciousness, I began to experience a basic human need - the need to urinate. (Robyn loves to tell this story.) Apparently, I did not want to urinate all over myself so I kept pointing at my groin area. No matter how many times Robyn told me it was okay to urinate, my brain did not comprehend that a catheter had been inserted into my penis.

According to Robyn, the incessant pointing at my crotch continued intermittently for hours until the catheter was removed later that night.

Taking Inventory Of The Situation

It was now about nine-thirty in the evening. The day had been a marathon for myself and my family. There was great news. I was alive. I was intact. The heart was pumping away and my new valves were opening and closing properly.

I was fixed.

It was now time for my family to return to their respective homes. It was also time for me to sleep. One-by-one, Doug, Monica, Jerry, Judy, Donna and Sylvia said their good-byes.

I fell back to sleep quickly.

The next time I awoke, I felt something very new and very uncomfortable.

I began to feel a physical pain in my chest, specifically in my incision.

Chris, my head cardiac nurse, had warned me days before, "When you wake up, you will feel two things. First, you will feel like a train has run you over. Second, you will feel tubes all over you."

Chris was incredibly accurate with her prediction.

First, I took tube inventory. I looked down and around. There were still five tubes connected to my body – two chest tubes, a central line in my neck, the intravenous drip and the catheter.

Tubes and wires monitoring my vital signs were everywhere.

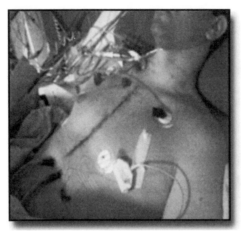

Picture Of Adam In The Intensive Care Unit
(Source: Robyn Pick)

Then, I took pain inventory. I could feel pain radiating from the incision. I was not moving. I was not doing anything. Yet, the pain was severe.

I had experienced worse – broken bones and compressed vertebra on the soccer field, the football field, and the tennis court. But, it had been awhile.

I then looked down to my chest.

There, I would see a bloody nine-inch scar that started at the tip of my chest plate and extended down my body to the top of my stomach. It was impressive. I had a 'zipper' as they called it. This was somewhat dislocating.

I now had permanent evidence of the life-altering operation that I did not remember.

Another Angel Appears

As the night progressed, the pain continued. At one point, I remember calling out for help. I could not remember the name of the ICU nurse. I simply remember asking loudly for help.

Then, I heard a familiar voice.

It was Robyn.

She chose to stay with me that first night in the intensive care unit.

For the next eight hours, she was my guardian angel.

If I needed more pain medication, she would negotiate the terms with Blythe. If I needed a more comfortable pillow, she would take care of it. If I needed someone to talk to, she would listen.

There are no words to explain what she did that night. She was angelic.

Throughout the night, a pattern developed.

I would awake, complain, and then go back to sleep.

This pattern would repeat itself over and over.

I would awake, complain and then go back to sleep.

Each time, Robyn would rise from the wooden chair (that she was using as a bed) and immediately comfort me.

In the middle of the night, however, I broke the pattern.

I awoke.

I did not complain.

Instead, I looked over at Robyn.

There, in her wooden chair, in the corner of the ICU room, Robyn sat alone with one eye open and one eye closed.

Even as she slept, my angel watched over me.

12

The Day After Surgery

In this chapter, you will:
- Understand what happens the day after your operation.
- Begin to learn more about heart valve surgery recovery.
- Review survey results specific to heart valve surgery recovery.

When I awoke the morning after surgery, I was hungry. The intravenous drip may have been replenishing my fluids but I needed to replenish my tummy.

Within seconds of sharing my hunger with the new ICU nurse, a menu fell into my two hands. (I believe the ICU nurse viewed my hunger as a very good sign.)

My eyes slowly scrolled the menu. I was impressed. The hospital had a great selection of food to choose from. I could order eggs, pancakes, fruit and more. The menu was four-pages long.

I found a personal favorite, oatmeal, on the second page and ordered it.

Getting Out Of Bed

As my room service order was working its way through the hospital, the ICU nurse asked me if I would like to eat my oatmeal sitting down on a chair outside my bed.

I think what she was really saying went something like this, "Adam, we know you have just had major surgery and we know you have been in bed for almost twenty four hours. However, we would like to encourage you to get out of bed so that your fear of life outside of your bed does not mature. Plus, we believe that movement will help your recovery."

I responded with, "Sure." This actually translated into, "I'm scared as hell to get out of this bed and experience the pain of my broken sternum and stitched heart, but I'm willing to give it a try."

The nurse shuffled the covers off my legs. Then, she adjusted the medical devices to my right side so that I would have an unobstructed walkway to the chair on the opposite side of the room.

She supported my arm and shoulder. I swiveled my legs off the bed. And then, on the count of three, I was on my feet again.

I let out an "Oh my god!" as my neurons comprehended the pain.

I did not panic.

I did not cry.

I focused on my goal.

I would walk to the chair on the other side of the room. I would eat my oatmeal. I would push myself to recover as fast as possible.

Similar to a newborn baby, my first steps were wobbly and uncalculated. To the outside observer, I would be judged as a drunk or a Frankenstein impersonator.

Seven steps later, I was being guided down into the orange chair.

"Good job Adam," I thought to myself.

The oatmeal arrived.

My mom and Aunt Sylvia arrived during breakfast. We enjoyed my morning success together.

My First Walk

As I told my family and doctors prior to the surgery, "Push me. Even if I don't want to do something, encourage me. I want this recovery to happen faster than slower."

Once I finished the oatmeal, the nurse asked me if I would like to go back to bed. While I could have returned to the bed, I wanted to better understand my surroundings and re-energize my legs.

I remember asking the nurse timidly, "Can I go for a walk?"

She responded that it would be okay but not to overdue it. We gathered up my tubes and headed out of my room onto the ICU floor. I took no more than twenty steps before I realized that I was tired and ready to return to bed. We walked back to my bed and I gingerly prepared for another dose of pain as I got back in bed.

 Getting in and out of bed would be one of the most uncomfortable activities of the following four weeks. Prior to heart surgery, I never had a problem with it. Now, that my chest was not yet healed, it was painful.

Even with the chest pain, I felt great. I had two major accomplishments that morning. I got up from bed and I went on my first walk.

The Spirometer

As I got back in bed and relaxed, I began to notice a different type of pain. It hurt when I breathed in. Each time I breathed in, I felt a little pinch in my lungs. To accommodate the pain, I began taking smaller breaths. That helped.

An hour or so later, Dave, a respiratory therapist, entered my room to check-up on me. I immediately questioned him about this breathing pain.

Dave asked me, "Have you been keeping up with your incentive spirometer?"

"Incentive spirometer?" I thought to myself, "What the heck is an incentive spirometer?"

The therapist then pointed to my bedside table where I saw an odd-looking breathing contraption that rekindled a memory.

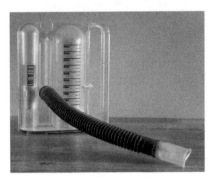

Incentive Spirometer

"Oh yeah," I thought to myself, "I remember that thing."

I had used the spirometer at some point during the night.

The therapist reached over and handed me the breathing apparatus. I lifted the mouthpiece to my lips and promptly blew into it as hard as I could.

"No!" the respiratory therapist exclaimed, "No, no, no. Let's start from the beginning."

Thankfully, Dave began to educate me.

"It is completely normal to have some pain when you inhale after surgery," he explained. "Naturally, most patients handle this by taking in small, shallow breaths. While that may seem like a good idea, it really isn't. The problem is, if you take shallow breaths for too long, the little air sacks in your lungs (the alveoli) start to collapse. That's bad."

"When the alveoli collapse," Dave continued, "They don't work. Breathing becomes harder. Even worse, collapsed alveoli can't defend themselves from bacteria. Your lungs may become infected and pneumonia will set in."

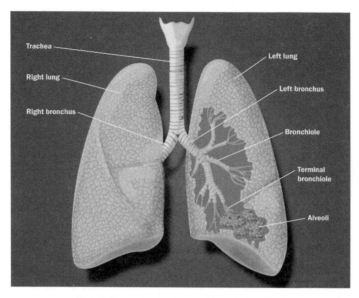

Alveoli Shown In Anatomy of Respiratory Tract

"So what can I do?" I asked.

"The key to preventing that problem is simple. Take in a deep, slow breath to the top of your lungs and hold it for five seconds. Pretend you are in a swimming pool and you are going to dunk your head underwater for five seconds."

I followed his instructions and took in the deepest breath I could, though it did hurt a bit. I held it for five seconds and let it out naturally.

"Perfect!" Dave exclaimed. "That's really all you need to do. As long as you do that throughout the day - about ten times an hour - you should be fine.

Then, the therapist pointed to the spirometer.

"Now, we are going to use the incentive spirometer," he said. "This time, do the exact same thing you just did. But, when you take that slow, deep breath, suck in through the mouthpiece. This device shows you two things. First, it shows how big your breath is. Secondly, it shows if you are breathing too fast. That's all."

As I took a slow, deep breath in, the plastic indicator went up, up, up. Then, I held my breath for five seconds. The indicator began to drop.

"Don't worry about that," the therapist continued, "The indicator starts falling as soon as you stop breathing in. Just note the level at which the indicator reached its peak. You did perfect."

"You do not have to use the spirometer," Dave continued, "Some people do better with it - usually the competitive types. They always want to beat their highest score, and this motivates them to take bigger breaths. That's good. But, the important thing is that you regularly take slow, big breaths and hold it for five seconds. Whether you do it on your own or through the spirometer, I don't really care. Just do it about ten times an hour when you are awake. I don't want you to get pneumonia. I'm sure you are eager to get home again."

"Yep. I'm not a fan of pneumonia," I replied. "So, I'll make sure to follow your instructions. Thanks!"

"One last thing," the therapist cautioned as he prepared to leave the room. "It would be really bad if you caught a cold or flu right now. So, it's probably best to not let anyone else use the spirometer until you are all healed up."

The incentive spirometer became one of my best friends over the next few weeks. I would take in big, slow breaths and monitor my improvement. Sometimes I would practice without it, but usually I would want to see how high I could lift the indicator. I guess I'm one of those competitive types.

Leaving The Intensive Care Unit

The rest of that first day after surgery was rather calm. My family came to visit.

At four o'clock in the afternoon, we learned that I was ready to leave the intensive care unit. The doctors and nurses told me that my heart was doing well and that my vital signs were normal.

My mom and Aunt Sylvia gathered my personal belongings. My nurse gathered my chest tubes, the spirometer and the drip. I slowly got out of bed and sat down in the wheelchair that was waiting for me. The nurse pushed, the wheels moved and a few seconds later I was on my way to room 550.

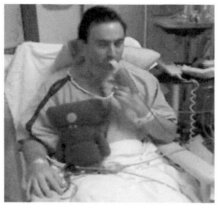

Adam Leaving The Intensive Care Unit
(Source: Robyn Pick)

Considering the unique nature of each patient case, I recently asked several patients the question, *"How long were you in the intensive care unit?"* Here are some of their responses:

- Geoff said, "I was in the I.C.U. (for a minimally invasive mitral valve repair) for 16 hours. The big thing they pushed was walking. I started at 8am the next morning. By the way, my 1 year anniversary was Wednesday!"

- Terry said, "After mitral valve repair and maze procedure, I was in the ICU for two days - lots and lots of tubes and IV's, but don't remember much else. My family was allowed almost unlimited visitation, and my husband stayed in the room with me - all rooms, even in the ICU, were private - and my husband tells me the nursing care was superb. So, don't worry. You get moved out when you are ready. Everyone is different!"

- Linda said, "I was in ICU for 7 days but I got pneumonia and my lungs collapsed so they kept me asleep and on a ventilator."

- Joan said, "I had my aortic valve replaced on Februrary 28, 2009. It was a 9am surgery and my husband tells me I got to the ICU about 2pm. I have no recollection of the next 12 hours including the removal of the breathing tube (thankfully). I was moved to the cardiac care unit at 4pm the next day, so 26 hours in ICU. Good Luck!"

13

The Final Days In The Hospital

In this chapter, you will:
- Learn what to expect after leaving the intensive care unit.
- Read about life in the hospital as a heart surgery patient.
- Get inspired by our *third* heart valve surgery success story.

I must admit, there was a sense of relief when I left the intensive care unit. The past two months had been a very anxious time. Now, it truly felt like the worst was behind me.

The surgery was over. The early indicators suggested that there was no regurgitation in my valves. While I was experiencing *muscular-skeletal* discomfort, I was told it would go away in six to eight weeks.

As I entered room 550, I immediately noticed the balloons and flowers that were delivered to the hospital for me. It felt great to physically see the support of my friends, family and co-workers.

Soon enough, the mood in the room elevated when my brother, Doug, surprised us all with a humongous order of food from my favorite delicatessen, Jerry's World Famous Deli. Although I was still dazed and tired, the smiles within my hospital room were memorable.

The Physical Discomfort

While I was mentally thrilled with my progress, my body was adjusting to the invasive procedure that fixed my heart. My incision and chest area continued to throb in pain. And, my lungs, even with my consistent use of the spirometer, hurt.

To help with the pain, the nurses offered me a number of pain relievers including Tylenol, Advil and Vicodin. Given the extreme nature of the discomfort, I opted for the Vicodin. Every four hours, I was entitled to two Vicodin.

A Good Night's Sleep

Considering I was no longer in the intensive care unit, I expected the second night in the hospital to be filled with uninterrupted sleep. To enhance that possibility, Nurse Matthew provided me with a sleeping pill called Halcion.

I woke up later that night in a cold sweat. When I awoke, I was alone. Unlike the intensive care unit, there were no nurses assigned to just me.

Instead, each nurse was responsible for a few patients. I reached for my phone and contacted the central, nursing station on the floor. It must have been two o'clock in the morning.

Nurse Matthew quickly appeared and explained that my night-sweat was normal, that it was nothing to be alarmed about. As he talked me down, the Halcion again took hold of my brain and I returned to sleep.

My Daily Activities Normalize

Over the next three days, my activities in the hospital would normalize. I developed a set pattern of activities that consisted of the following:

- Walking around the hospital floor
- Using the spirometer
- Ordering room service
- Napping twice daily
- Watching television
- Spending time with my family

That's really all I did during my final three days in the hospital. I would not say that I was bored in the hospital. I was more dazed and tired.

I would later learn that the general anesthetic administered during my surgery has a significant half-life. It is believed by many that the effects of general anesthesia can be felt for days, weeks and even months after surgery.

For Female Patients... Bra Use After Surgery?

For many women, a common concern following surgery relates to breast support. In fact, I just received a question from Vicki that reads, "What about a bra? I have heavy breasts and I can see that this could be a problem after valve surgery. I was just wondering how soon after surgery will I be able to wear a bra? Does anyone have any suggestions about this?"

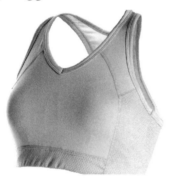

To help Vicki, I asked several female patients to provide their thoughts on this topic:

• Cynthia said, "My mom just had surgery. She is 84 and has had a radical mastectomy, so she needs to wear a bra and a prosthesis. She has been wearing both comfortably ever since her discharge, 10 days after surgery. She has never indicated that it was a problem. I was her primary caregiver for three weeks afterwards and the only issue with the bra was getting some help to hook it behind her. She didn't even need help all the time, just some days."

• Becca said, "I am three weeks post surgery, and I was able to wear a regular bra two weeks after surgery. I probably could have worn one earlier, but didn't try to! I am not very large in that area, so support was a non-issue! I usually wear stretchy sports bras, but found they were a little hard to pull on with sore chest muscles, so I went with a standard bra."

• Joanne said, "I had valve repair 5 months ago. My surgeon told me to wear a bra all the time - for the first few weeks. So I wore a somewhat loose sports-type bra. It felt good... Like an added support layer holding my chest together - which you totally don't need to worry about, but I did anyways. If you can get a bra that fastens in back, that's even better. Because lifting your arms can be a bit uncomfortable for a while."

- Carol said, "Explain your concerns to your surgeon before surgery. You are not the first woman to have this problem. **Don't be surprised if you wake up with a post-op bra on!** There have been documented studies which conclude that post-op bras actually reduce the incidence of pulling on the suture line, thus controlling pain better and promoting healing sooner."

Highlights Of Hospital Life

During my last three days in the hospital, there were a few experiences and activities that I will highlight for you now:

- **X-rays.** Each morning, I would be taken to radiology for an x-ray.

- **Doctor rounds.** The doctors would make their rounds once a day. USC is a teaching university, so it was very interesting to see the academic nature of my case discussed among the attending physicians, residents and interns.

- **Respiration therapy.** As the pain in my lungs continued for the first forty-eight hours after surgery, I was given respiration therapy every four hours starting on my third day in the hospital. The therapy consisted of inhaling and exhaling a steroid for fifteen minutes.

- **Chest tubes.** On the fourth day in the hospital, my chest tubes were finally removed from my body. Although the physical act of removing the tubes from my upper body stung somewhat, it felt amazing once they were successfully removed.

- **Shower.** On the fifth day in the hospital, I took my first and only shower in the hospital. Robyn took me into the shower, removed my clothes and washed me from head to toe. It felt amazing.

- **Bowel movement.** It was not until my fifth day in the hospital, that I successfully completed my first, post-operative bowel movement.

- **Drugs.** My dependence on medication for physical relief and sleep continued throughout my stay in the hospital. At one point, Nurse Matthew asked me if I had been a heavy user of narcotics in the past. According to the nurse, my intake of drugs was somewhat concerning. I assured him that prior to heart valve surgery, I had never even seen a narcotic.

Leaving The Hospital – Christmas Day, 2005

Although Dr. Darbinian informed me that I was medically ready to leave the hospital on the fourth day, I chose to stay one extra day to be safe.

I woke up on Christmas morning ready to experience a great present.

I was going home.

My brother was scheduled to pick me up at one thirty in the afternoon. Robyn and I did our normal routine before the pick-up. We ordered room service. We walked around the ward. We watched television. We packed up my things and dressed me in a freshly washed pair of pajamas.

About one half-hour before Doug arrived to take me home, my nurse sat me down and provided me with some basic guidelines for post-operative care and recovery.

Those guidelines were referenced in a twenty-page hand-out which we reviewed together.

The most important points he noted were:

- Do not lift anything greater than five pounds for the first four weeks.
- Do not drive a car for the first six weeks.
- Do not overexert yourself.
- Get plenty of rest.

When we finished the discussion, he gave me a set of prescriptions that included Vicodin and Halcion. The nurse also told me it was critical that I purchase Peri-Colace. Peri-Colace is an over-the-counter stool softener/stimulant laxative used in the treatment of occasional constipation (irregularity) often caused by pain medications like Vicodin.

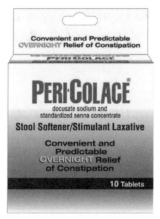

Peri Colace Stool Softener
(Source: Purdue Pharma, LLC)

I then signed some discharge paperwork.

A wheelchair arrived outside of my room about five minutes later.

During my final wheelchair ride, I said several *'goodbyes'* and *'thank yous'* to the nurses and doctors on the floor.

Four days after heart valve surgery, I was leaving USC medical center with a new heart and a second chance at life.

Heart Valve Surgery Success Story - Veronika Meyer
Mountain Climber Phenomena

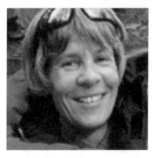

The story of Veronika Meyer is extraordinary. A heart valve replacement recipient at age forty-six, Veronika has a unique mountain climbing hobby. Actually, mountain climbing is more than a hobby for Veronika. It's more of an obsession for the scientist from St. Gallen, Switzerland.

Since receiving a St. Jude Medical mechanical heart valve in 1997, Veronika Meyer's mountain climbing accomplishments include the ascent of Mount McKinley, the highest mountain in North America, and Aconcagua, the highest peak of both the Americas.

In 2003, Veronika Meyer attempted the ultimate mountain climbing challenge - Mount Everest. Unfortunately, Veronika's first attempt was not a success. Veronika was forced to turn back just below the famous Second Step landmark because of a heavy storm.

Although disappointed, Veronika was pleased to have climbed to 8,600 meters or 28,215 feet—her "personal best" altitude.

Then, in 2005, Veronika made her second attempt to summit Mount Everest, but had to turn back at 7800 meters because of unpredictable weather conditions. Although two members of Veronika's team reached the peak, a third member tragically died during that expedition.

Veronika experienced three failed attempts to climb to the top of the world, located at 8,850 meters (29,035 feet) above sea level.

However, in 2007, on her fourth attempt, Veronika conquered Mount Everest. By all known accounts, Veronika Meyer is the first mountain climber implanted with a mechanical heart valve to successfully ascend Everest.

"Conditions were excellent this year with a lot of snow, but in addition, all of us were strong," Meyer said.

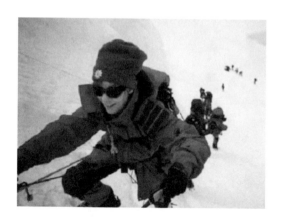

Since New Zealander Edmund Hillary and Sherpa Tenzing Norgay first reached Everest in 1953, about 2,000 climbers have scaled the mountain. Another 205 people have died on its dangerous slopes.

"Veronika's amazing accomplishment should offer inspiration to millions of heart-valve patients around the world," said George Fazio, president of St. Jude's cardiovascular division. "Despite living with a heart condition for many years, she has refused to accept limits and has pursued her goals with tremendous courage and determination."

PART IV
RECOVERING FROM
VALVE SURGERY

chapter

14

Everybody's Recovery Is Different

In this chapter, you will:
- Understand that recovering from heart valve surgery is a personal process.
- Learn that the rate of the recovery will vary.

One of the questions I had specific to heart valve surgery was, "How long will it take to recover from the operation?"

People ask this question for several different reasons. Some people want to know how long they will need to be away from work. Some people want to know how long they will need medical care when they return from the hospital. Other people want to know how long they might be in physical discomfort as a result of the surgery.

"So, How Long Does It Take To Recover?"

The first time I searched the Internet, looking for answers to this question, I found several resources which stated that the average recovery time from heart valve surgery was eight to twelve weeks. That seemed like a pretty significant amount of time. So, I decided to double-check with my surgeon.

When I asked Dr. Starnes that question, he said, "Adam, you're a young guy. I think you are going to snap back in no time."

While that response made me feel good, Dr. Starnes did not exactly answer the question.

I then asked some former patients that I met online at www.valvereplacement. com.

Again, I was confused by the variance in recovery times. Some patients were back at work in five weeks. Other patients were out of work for several months.

As I would continue to learn during my recovery, the rate of healing is different for each person that has heart valve surgery. *There is no set period of time that you should use as a standardized benchmark.*

As you will read in later chapters, my recovery did not occur in eight to twelve weeks. I did not 'snap back' during my recovery. Rather, it was a very challenging process that involved several mental and physical obstacles.

I am telling you this now, at the beginning of 'Part IV - The Recovery', to emphasize this overlooked and often mismanaged element of cardiac surgery recovery.

Again, everyone recovers from heart valve surgery at a different rate. *There is no pre-defined recovery time.*

Since my surgery, I have spoken with many valve repair and valve replacement patients. In hearing their stories, I learned over-and-over again, that the time to recover varies based upon the procedure, the body and its ability to heal.

The recovery can be very frustrating. *My own personal recovery from heart valve surgery was filled with frustration, confusion, anger, sorrow and depression.*

I remember one night, when I looked at Robyn, my wife, and said, "My mind and body are no longer one. I am not recovering fast enough."

She then presented me with one of the greatest pieces of advice I received during my recovery. She said to me, "Adam, you're just going to have to hurry up and wait. I know it is going to be hard for you. But, you have no choice."

I smiled. I got it. She was right. I had no choice. I had no way to speed up my healing. At times, Robyn is just genius.

However, as I would also learn, there are a number of mental and physical actions you can take to stimulate the healing process. These recovery tips can also help you avoid some of the common pitfalls that might arise during your healing.

Survey Results – Recovering From Heart Valve Surgery

I was very curious to know what other patients felt about their recovery. So, I coordinated a survey with many former, heart valve surgery patients.

As you have already seen, I asked a number of questions during that survey. Here are survey results for questions specific to heart valve surgery recovery.

The first question I asked was very straightforward.

I asked the respondents to complete the following statement, "My recovery from heart valve surgery was _____." The possible answers provided to the respondents were: *easier than I expected, about what I expected or more difficult than I expected.*

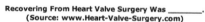
Recovering From Heart Valve Surgery Was _____.
(Source: www.Heart-Valve-Surgery.com)

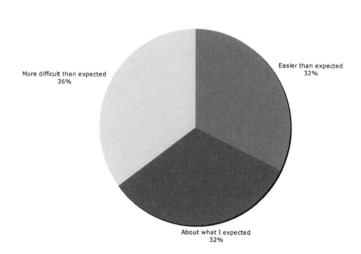

More difficult than expected
36%

Easier than expected
32%

About what I expected
32%

The survey results were very interesting! As you can see, most survey participants said that recovery from heart valve surgery was *more difficult than expected (36%)*.

However, while the majority of respondents noted that recovering from heart valve surgery was more difficult than expected, it was only by a slight margin compared to the other two responses. In fact, it was very encouraging to see that 32% of respondents believed that heart valve surgery recovery was easier than expected.

Next, I asked a question directly to those patients who returned to work following their heart valve operation. The question I asked was, "How long did it take you to return to work following heart valve surgery?"

As you can see, there is a wide range of responses to this question.

A number of factors could have influenced these results. The *type* of valve surgery could have influenced these results (open heart surgery versus minimally invasive robotic surgery). Also, whether or not the patient experienced any complications following surgery could have influenced the survey results.

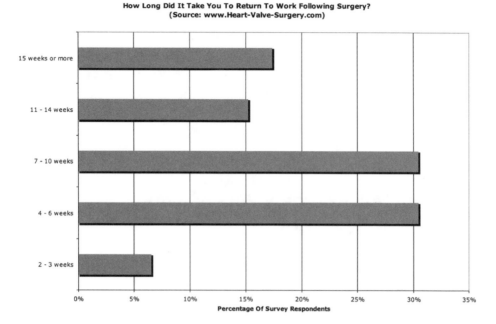

How Long Did It Take You To Return To Work Following Surgery?
(Source: www.Heart-Valve-Surgery.com)

Still, the most common timeframe for patients returning to work was between four and ten weeks.

Again, as previously stated and restated in this chapter, everybody's recovery rate will be different.

To this point, I recently posted a blog that asked the question, *"When were you 100% recovered?"* Here are some of the responses to that question:

- Shelby said, "I was fully recovered about six months after surgery. The first three months showed the greatest improvement... The next three months, I experienced a more gradual return to normality."

- Kathy said, "At 16 months post-op I am just beginning to really feel like myself. I had some complications with my aortic valve replacement."

- Todd said, "I am 43 and had my mitral valve replaced on April 4, 2009. Now it's June 2 and I feel about 80-85%."

- Tom said, "I am now 6 months from mitral valve repair and single bypass. I feel like I am at 90%. The problem has been the healing of my split sternum. I am, however, playing golf again and walking 18 holes. I am 75 years old."

You can view all of the responses to the question, *"When were you 100% recovered?"* at the following link - http://www.heart-valve-surgery.com/heart-surgery-blog/2009/06/02/recovery-time/.

Former Valve Surgery Patient Quote: Adrienne de Burgos (Quebec)

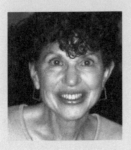

"Don't get discouraged the first few days after surgery. It is normal to feel very weak and to feel nauseous at the beginning. Just let people help you at the beginning and you will see progress each day."

chapter

15

Coming Home From The Hospital

In this chapter, you will:
- Know what to expect as you return home from the hospital.
- Learn some tips and tricks to help your early recovery.

I will never forget leaving the hospital. After five long days in the cardiothoracic ward at USC, I experienced both excitement and fear as the nurse wheeled me into the fresh air of Los Angeles.

I was excited to go home. I was excited the surgery was over. I was excited that my heart was doing great.

I was excited to move on with my life. I was excited to recover.

On the other hand, I was afraid. I was afraid that something might go wrong. I was afraid that my heart might fail. I was afraid that I would not have a nurse or doctor on call should something negative happen.

That was a very curious moment when I stood up from the wheelchair.

I was happy and sad together.

As we drove the fifteen miles home on Christmas Day, I thought about all that had happened during the past five days.

Then I thought about all that had occurred during the past two months. From Dr. Bad Bedside Manner to my collapse in Europe. From finding Dr. Starnes to dealing with the insurance company. From getting shaved in the pre-op room to walking in the intensive care unit.

I do not think anyone saw, but I cried for the majority of the ride home.

"It's over," I thought to myself. "It really is over."

Little did I know, it was not over.

In fact, the biggest challenge specific to my heart valve surgery had just begun. That challenge was my recovery.

Getting In And Out Of Bed

Upon arrival at my home, it did not take long for me to realize that I was tired and ready for a nap. I entered my bedroom and, with the help of my brother, laid down on my bed.

My chest radiated a severe pain as I laid flat for the first time in five days. This was a new experience. This was an experience I would not forget any time soon.

While it was uncomfortable and painful getting into bed that day, I would later find out that it would be equally as painful getting out of bed. The pain was situated around and within the incision.

 I would later learn that many patients use a recliner during their early recovery from heart surgery. A recliner can minimize the pressure on the broken sternum and the sternal wires as the patient assumes a resting position.

In a recent discussion with Max, an aortic valve replacement patient, he noted, "My wife and I bought a recliner for the specific purpose of helping with my recovery. If I did not have it, I don't know how I would have made it through the first 3 weeks at home after surgery."

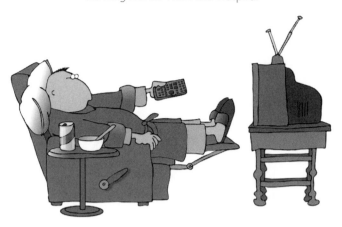

Other patients had the following to say about recliner use after surgery:

- Bruce said, "I personally would have been lost without a recliner following my surgery. I would call it a must. However, make sure it has a handle."

- Debbi said, "I did use a recliner in addition to my bed (propped up with lots of pillows). I found having a change of position helpful. The discomfort in my shoulders after surgery made staying in one position for long periods quite uncomfortable."

- Tim said, "I rented a power recliner for a month... I was glad I did! It was easy getting into the sleeping position and the recliner helped push me out. I had the recliner delivered BEFORE my surgery so it was waiting for me when I came home. I put a TV tray right next to the recliner to hold all my necessities - remote, pills, drink, etc."

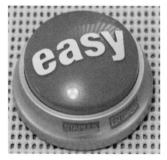

As I prepared to take my first nap, my brother handed me an electronic toy from Staples, the office products store. He said, "When you need me, just press this button. It will make a loud noise and I'll know you're awake."

It was an ingenious idea. I did not have the energy to yell through closed doors. It made perfect sense – almost like a bell to ring for a butler. However, I'm not rich and he was not my butler.

I tested it right there and then. When I pressed the button, an electronics voice beckoned, "That was easy!" I laughed. If only the people at Staples knew how we were using their company toy.

Getting To Know Your Pharmacist

I would sleep for two hours. When I awoke, I pressed the Staples button.

Robyn entered the room. I had to go to the bathroom but did not want to leave the comfort of my bed. Robyn helped me urinate into the plastic jar that we brought home from the hospital.

As I lay in bed, I noticed that the pain in my chest was returning. It had been almost four hours since my last dose of Vicodin. It was time to take those two *wonderful* pills again. Thankfully, Robyn had gone to the Rite-Aid during my nap. My prescriptions were filled.

While there, Robyn befriended Betty, a pharmacist who had been working for Rite-Aid for over twenty years. Our relationship with Betty would grow over the next few months considering our frequent visits to the pharmacy.

 Before entering the hospital for your surgery, make sure you know the phone numbers of your local pharmacy. You should also know the phone number of the closest <u>twenty-four hour</u> pharmacy as well.

In the hospital I learned that Vicodin really helped manage my pain. Twenty minutes after taking these miracle pills, my chest pain would downgrade from throbbing discomfort to barely noticeable.

Taking Short Walks

During my first few days at home, I found that taking short walks was very helpful.

I found these walks helpful for two key reasons. First, it just felt good to be moving. I estimate that during my five days in the hospital, I was in bed ninety-five percent of the time. I needed to re-animate my life. I needed to move. I needed to get my heart rate up. I needed to re-experience the freedom of life outside of a bed.

The second reason I found walking helpful was that I could monitor my progress by the length of the walk. For example, when Robyn and I took that first walk after my return from the hospital, I only made it to the end of my driveway and back. In total, it could not have been more than one hundred feet.

We walked slowly. Let me rephrase that... We walked *very* slowly. I was still in my robe and slippers as we walked together outside. Again, it was Christmas Day. I could only imagine what my neighbors must have been thinking.

The next time we walked, however, I could make it to the end of my driveway and back two times. Although it was only a distance of two hundred feet, it felt great to experience physical progress.

 Taking short walks provided me with two key benefits during the early phase of my recovery – physical and emotional progress.

The short walks also provided me with an emotional boost. Not only was I experiencing physical advances, but the short walks forced me to get out of bed, to breathe fresh air and to feel the sun on my face. I always felt inspired after a walk even though it was challenging to move during those first few days back from the hospital.

Reach Out To Your Support Group

Earlier in this book, I noted that your support group would be critical to your recovery. Now that you are home from the hospital, you will really understand why.

As you adjust to being home, you will be confronted by your physical limitations. For example, it might be challenging to open the refrigerator door because of your chest pain. You might also have a challenge taking a shower. There were many challenges that I faced due to my physical limitations.

When I returned from the hospital, I remember feeling that *I might break* if I did something requiring lifting, pulling or pushing. That feeling was most prominent during the following activities:

- Opening the refrigerator
- Putting on my clothes
- Tying my shoes
- Lifting anything
- Opening the car door
- Putting on my seat belt
- Getting out of bed
- Taking a shower

The reality was... I was not going to break from these actions. Still, it was very helpful to have my mom, my brother, my sister or my dad there to help and encourage me.

I heard that the first two weeks after surgery would be quite uncomfortable. Therefore, I communicated with my friends and family that I would like to have someone with me each day for the first fourteen days after my return from the hospital. My support group agreed to this request and I prepared a schedule. I then emailed it to everyone on the list.

 Having someone from my support group with me each day during the first two weeks after surgery was very helpful for my physical and emotional well-being.

Again, communication with your support group is critical. I highly encourage you to ask your friends and family to spend time with you during the initial part of your recovery.

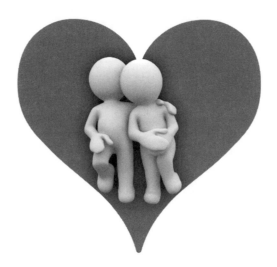

It's amazing when I look back and think about all the fun we had. My brother, Doug, showed me how to make his one-of-a-kind egg salad. My sister planted lavender and gardenias in the front yard. My mom and I went on several walks. My dad and I had breakfasts together. My friends, Rob and Rachel, visited me from Virginia and Chicago. I am truly blessed that my support group rallied around me like they did!

Follow-Up Doctor Visits With The Cardiologist

Two weeks after surgery, my recovery was slowly coming along. I was still sleeping a lot. I started to notice that the little things that used to bother me (putting on a t-shirt) didn't bother me so much. I was showering on my own and I was taking short walks three times each day. My mom and I even walked along the beach one day.

I saw Dr. Rosin, my cardiologist, during the second week after my surgery. Dr. Rosin took a listen to my heart and said, "Excellent. Your heart sounds great. I'll see you in a month for a follow-up echo."

I then told Dr. Rosin that I was still experiencing severe chest pain and my lungs continued to pinch when I breathed. Dr. Rosin informed me that chest pain was typical and that I should give it time. He explained that the heart was doing great and the other *muscular-skeletal* issues would work themselves out as my body healed.

As for the breathing pain, Dr. Rosin asked me, "Are you still using the spirometer?"

I said, "No."

"There ya go," Dr. Rosin smiled, "You've got a little bit of fluid in your lungs. Start blowing on that spirometer and the breathing pain will go away in two days."

The former USC football player turned cardiologist, then reached out and gently pulled back the skin around my eyelids. "Hmmm. You've got *anemia*," Dr. Rosin said, "In addition to the spirometer blowing, get some iron in your system. Eat some meat or go buy some chopped liver."

Dr. Rosin was right. A few days after using the spirometer the pain in my sides was gone and color was returning to my skin. I was no longer pale from the anemia. I must have eaten two pounds of chopped liver that week.

Follow-Up Doctor Visits With The Surgeon

During my third week after surgery, I went to see Dr. Starnes, my surgeon. When Dr. Starnes entered the examination room, a unique wave of emotions came over me and I burst into tears. I'm not sure how to explain it, but I had some special connection with this surgical wizard that just made me feel very good, very comfortable, and now that my heart was fixed, very indebted.

Truth be known, I actually got down on my hands and knees to show my appreciation. He quickly lifted me up.

Dr. Starnes wasted no time and positioned me on the examination table while he listened to my heart with his stethoscope.

He looked up, smiled and said, "You sound just perfect." Dr. Starnes then told me, "The recovery is going to really pick-up in the next few weeks. You are going to be feeling great."

In a very strange conversation that followed, Dr. Starnes then told me about my diseased heart valve. I will never forget what he said about the valve.

"Adam," Dr. Starnes said, "Your valve was very sick, very calcified. It was in *really* bad shape. It's a good thing we got it out of there when we did."

The tears continued as I thought about what my calcified valve might have looked like. I wanted to see it but I did not have the energy to ask.

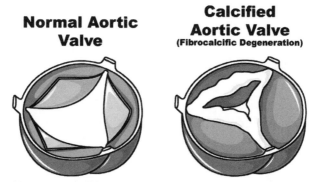

Normal and Calcified Heart Valves (Source: Servier International)

Regarding my ongoing chest-pain, Dr. Starnes said that my chest would need another few weeks to heal and that I should keep taking the pain meds as needed. "You should be able to drive in a few more weeks. Take care Adam. I'll see you next December for the one year check-up."

Before leaving, I asked Dr. Starnes if his other patients were using Mederma. He knew nothing about the product. Mederma is a topical care product (gel) for scars used after surgery, accidents, injuries, burns, acne, and stretch marks.

I showed him the product. Dr. Starnes read the ingredients and said, "This looks good. I do not see any reason why you shouldn't use it."

He smiled. We shook hands. Dr. Starnes was moving on to the next patient.

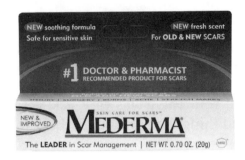

Mederma Skin Care Product
(Source: Merz)

My Pain Medication Consumption Raises Eyebrows

After Dr. Starnes left the room, I spoke with Chris, his head nurse. I told Chris that I was running low on Vicodin and that I needed another prescription.

She looked at me in an *odd way* and curiously asked, "Are you still taking two pills every four hours?"

I nodded my head up and down.

Her left eyebrow lifted.

"And you *really* need all that medication?" Chris asked me.

I nodded my head up and down again.

"Alright. Let's start taking the dosage down to one pill every four hours," she said, "And, if you need to, supplement it with Advil or Motrin. I don't want you to get hooked on this stuff."

She wrote the prescription and my mother and I left USC Medical Center on San Pablo Road once again.

The Incision Shield For Discomfort

One product for incision discomfort to consider during early recovery is the Incision Shield. Simply worn around the neck, this light post-operative device spans the incision site and protects the incision while patients resume daily activities.

The Incision Shield is flexible and suitable for all patients recovering from heart valve surgery – both male or female. Ultimately, the Incision Shield helps patients minimize incision pain and enhance scar healing.

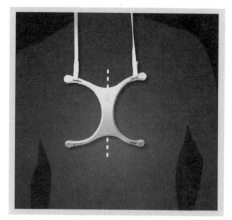

The Incision Shield
(Source: Incision Shield)

Several patients and surgeons have offered testimonials for this unique product:

- Doug Atkins, a heart surgery patient, said, "If you are going in for open heart surgery, I HIGHLY recommend the use of one of these Incision Shields. I used the shield for about 3 weeks after my surgery and it worked incredibly well! Definitely keeps clothing off of your incision... which is a wonderful thing!"

- Betty Marshall, a heart surgery patient, said, "The Incision Shield is wonderful. It fits wonderfully around my neck and has kept my clothing from irritating my incision."

- Dr. Thomas Williams, Jr., M.D., a cardiac surgeon, said, "I highly endorse the Incision Shield as an aid in pain control."

After speaking with the owners of Incision Shield, I was able to negotiate a 27% discount for readers of this book. If you would like to purchase this product, please visit **www.HeartSurgeryShield.com**.

16

Cardiac Depression

It was the third week of my recovery and everything seemed to be coming along nicely. Although I was experiencing a good deal of chest pain, I was feeling good enough that I even spent some time alone.

Spending Time Alone

Although I was alone, I was not independent. I still had a hard time doing many of the little things that I took for granted prior to my surgery.

For example, my incision hurt when I tried to open twist-off caps on drinks (water, orange juice). I also had a challenging time reaching into the back of the refrigerator to get food to make lunch and dinner.

I told Robyn and my mom about these challenges and they immediately came up with some thoughtful ideas to help.

- Before Robyn left for work in the morning, she would pre-open two or three drinks and then put the cap back on with a subtle twist so that I could open it easily when I was thirsty.

- As for food, everyone started bringing me ready-made food (salads, tuna, sandwiches, chopped liver, pastrami, chicken salad) and nutrition bars so I could eat or snack when I was hungry. You should have seen my refrigerator! It was stuffed with food.

As for daily activities, walking remained my passion. I was now walking around the block. Everyday I could walk a little bit further.

The Pain Becomes A Problem

Following my visit to Dr. Starnes' office, I took Nurse Chris' suggestion and cut back the amount of Vicodin from eight pills each day to four pills each day.

The impact of the dosage shift was immediate. Within hours of missing the second two-pill dose, pain was everywhere. The discomfort that previously radiated from my incision now stretched clear across my chest.

Again, at Nurse Chris' suggestion, I took a few Advil to help manage the pain.

No change. The discomfort continued.

I remember thinking to myself, "Oh my god! Is this what life is like without painkillers?" and "Have I been so doped up on Vicodin that I never truly experienced the actual pain that accompanied heart valve surgery?"

I called Uncle Marc. Marc Darrow is a well-known physician who owns a wonderful sports rehabilitation clinic in Santa Monica, California called Joint Rehab (www.1800rehab10.com). I told Marc about my situation and he told me to be *very* careful about Vicodin addiction. Although I did not know this when I started to take the pain medication, Vicodin is very addictive.

Marc also shared with me that it was still early in my recovery and that if I needed more Vicodin for the first six weeks or so, I should take it. Marc told me to call him if I needed more medication.

After our call, I immediately walked to the medicine cabinet and took another Vicodin. Twenty minutes later, I was relieved from the pain.

I decided to slowly wean myself off the Vicodin. I remember thinking, "I'm no addict!"

I crafted a personal plan to reduce my pain medication consumption.

"I'll slowly take the number of pain pills from eight per day to seven to six to five and so on over the next few weeks," I thought.

To help, I even created a chart to help me track the amount of pills I consumed on a hourly basis. I would mark the number of pills I took throughout the current, twenty-four hour period. Each night, I would review my progress with Robyn.

"What's Wrong With Me?"

It was during the fifth week of my recovery that I started to have some concern about my recovery. I was still in a lot of pain.

According to the Internet, most people were driving by their fourth week and getting ready to go back to work by their eighth week. I, on the other hand, was nowhere close to driving a car. Going back to work was the furthest thing from my mind.

I was also noticing an emotional shift in my behavior and attitude towards my health.

Since I began reducing my pain medication, I found myself crying more frequently. The smallest negative thought or negative feeling could set me off into a downward spiral that typically generated a rhetorical question that teased and taunted me.

That question was "What is wrong with me?"

Said differently, the question could also translate into, "What are they not telling me?" or "Am I going to be like this forever?" or "When is this going to stop?" and "Why is my recovery going so slow?"

This was not a fun time - for me or my family.

My emotions manifested themselves in my physical appearance. I walked slowly, dragging my feet. When I walked, I also rolled my shoulders forward and tucked my chest inward. My upper body conformed into a concave shape.

I was tired all the time.

I never wanted to leave the house.

And, worst of all, I was resigned to the possibility that I would get better.

Each day started to blur into the next. There was little progress to share with my family or friends. I was so depressed that I even stopped calling certain members of my support group. I got so tired of sounding like a broken record of complaints. This hurts. No, that hurts. This hurts.

"Just let me be in my misery," I thought to myself.

Then, my voice left me. In its place, appeared a cold, distant and fearful voice. I was monotone and lifeless. My voice was embarrassing. In fact, I did my best not to speak by selecting the least amount of words to convey a thought or feeling.

My frustration impacted the people around me. I was so removed from them. I sought refuge in my own dark space.

I entered cardiac depression in the sixth week following surgery.

Again, I thought, "What's wrong with me?"

Dealing With Cardiac Depression

My family desperately searched for a solution to my depression. While months ago they were searching for a surgeon, now they were searching for a cure to my depression.

Blame was placed on the drugs. My family's fingers pointed to the one thing that actually helped me with pain and sleep.

150

It was now seven weeks after my surgery and I was still taking four to five Vicodin each day. Plus, I was an insomniac again. So, I took Halcion each night to help me sleep.

Robyn was most aggressive. She threatened to throw-out all the pills in our house. We fought and fought and fought over my use, and supposed abuse, of the medication. She didn't understand why I still needed to take the drugs. I did my best to explain. She broke down in tears. Our frustration was shared.

To help her, my family and perhaps myself, I went cold turkey (stopped taking medication) on a Saturday in early February. I slept for two hours that night. The next morning, Robyn and I went to breakfast at Jerry's Deli in Marina Del Rey. It was chilly and wet outside.

As we sat in the maroon leather booth, I could not eat. I could not talk. I was cold. I felt nauseous. Then, I noticed a most peculiar movement in my body. My hands were shaking. I took a few Advil. The shaking continued. I took some more Advil. No help. More shaking.

"Is this what it feels like to be a drug addict?" I asked Robyn.

She assured me it would be okay.

"What's wrong with me?" the question returned once again.

Robyn could see the anxiety that appeared on my face. "It will be okay."

She was wrong that day. It wasn't okay.

I was angry and frustrated. My life was upside down. I wanted out of my body. I wanted relief. I wanted to be normal again. I wanted my life back. I wanted to be healthy. I wanted to stop shaking. I wanted to eat. I wanted to go to the gym. I wanted to swim. I wanted to surf.

And, then I realized...

I needed Vicodin...

I needed help.

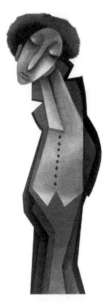

Research Spotlight:
Why Is Depression Common In Cardiac Patients?

Reports suggest that between 30% to 75% of patients report feeling anxious or depressed after heart surgery. Fortunately, a vast majority of patients who do suffer depression emotionally recover within six months. Still, for those patients who deal with overwhelming gloom, the postoperative weeks can seem intolerable.

"I think there is a significant incidence of acute postoperative depression, which uniformly resolves in a period of weeks," notes Dr. R. Scott Mitchell, professor of cardiovascular surgery at Stanford. "I think the cause is entirely unknown, but it could be the psychological effect of anticipating the surgery; the prolonged time under anesthesia, which is about four or five hours; or the results of the heart-lung machine."

Post-surgery cardiac depression can also be caused by a number of reasons including being worried that something is wrong, being afraid of dying, fearing that your recovery is problematic and being concerned about the success of your operation.

Reports suggest that depression after cardiac surgery appears to be increasing in frequency. In the opinion of some, this increase is directly related to the short hospital stays in which patients are discharged four or five days after the operation.

Years ago, patients would have ten to fourteen days in the hospital to assimilate their new reality, to accept their status as cardiac patients, and to digest what it means to them, their families and their lifestyles, according to Dr. Richard Fogoros, M.D. in *Why Is Depression So Common In Cardiac Patients*. In many cases, they would have received repeated instructions from medical personnel about their heart condition, and what they should be doing to improve their odds of symptom-free, long-term survival. So that, by the time they were sent home, many of them would have begun to regain a legitimate sense of control over their own fates and/or fears.

Today, the techniques of cardiac surgery have vastly improved. Accordingly, the odds of surviving heart valve surgery are much better today than they were a mere decade or two ago.

However, Dr. Fogoros reminds us that the rapid, patient transformation from the hospital to the 'real world' may elevate a new sense of fragile mortality. Sometimes, patients are only given a brief ten-to-fifteen page guide to teach them what to do and what not to do following surgery. Often times, no cardiac rehabilitation program is established for the patient.

For many people who have had bypass surgery, regaining emotional strength is a tougher challenge than recuperating physically.

In *Facing Up To Depression After A Bypass*, Randi Epstein suggests that rehabilitation specialists working with bypass patients have focused on rebuilding weakened muscles after surgery. But recently, cardiac specialists — nurses, doctors and psychologists — have begun to concentrate on the mental fatigue and overwhelming sadness that strikes many patients.

The Onset Of Cardiac Depression

At times, the patient may become depressed after returning home, even if there are no signs during hospitalization. According to Dr. Robert Matthews, a cardiologist in Los Angeles, California, the symptoms may be manifested as pain and fatigue, instead of, or in addition to, mental signs.

As I personally learned, it can take over a month for the impact of being a heart valve surgery patient to truly sink in. The uncertainties of your mobility and a quick return to work may cause additional worry to you and your family. These fears and changing emotions are normal and a natural reaction to the stress of the event, according to Dr. Fogoros.

 You will have good days and bad days. For the first few months after cardiac surgery, I felt like I was on a rollercoaster. Some days were amazing. I had vigor, energy and strength. Other days, however, I was achey, tired and resigned.

Most people, however start to feel better as time passes, as they get back into their usual routine and their anxiety starts to lessen.

What Are The Signs Of Cardiac Depression?

If you experience tiredness, irritability, loss of appetite, difficulty with sleeping, find it difficult to concentrate, feel tearful on a regular basis, lose interest in things you normally enjoy, or start to lose your temper easily, it may be a sign of depression, according to Healthy Place, an anxiety community (http://www.healthyplace.com).

Depression and anxiety can also cause physical symptoms, which are sometimes very similar to the symptoms of coronary heart disease, including tiredness, chest pain, breathlessness and palpitations. These symptoms may vary from day to day.

Experiencing difficulties with sexual activities after cardiac surgery may also cause anxiety. Returning to gentle sexual activity around three to four weeks after surgery is usually quite safe depending on your speed of recovery.

There may be loss of libido or impotence for men, which may be due to anxiety or depression, the chest discomfort after surgery, or because of certain medications such as beta-blockers or diuretics. If you think your medication may be affecting you in this way, or you have any concerns about restarting sexual activity, you should discuss it with your general practitioner, cardiologist, or cardiac rehabilitation nurse.

How To Manage Cardiac Depression?

It is important to discuss any problems with your doctor as they may be able to help you resolve your anxieties. If your anxiety or depression becomes severe, and there is no sign of improvement, you may need treatment from your doctor or a professional counselor.

Making your friends and family aware of the way you are feeling can help their understanding of your situation. **It can also be reassuring for you and your family to know that these problems are usually temporary.**

Dr. Matthews suggests in *Convalescent Depression After A Myocardial Infarction Or Heart Surgery* that the patient's family or "significant other" may require help to deal with the stress of the situation, which usually involves heightened responsibilities as well as care of an agitated patient. The crisis situation of the cardiac surgery and the resulting role changes and stresses can unleash emotional problems up to two years later and may have an adverse affect on relationships.

 Changing emotions such as feeling depressed, bad tempered, angry or guilty can strain even the closest of relationships and bottling up these feelings can lead to difficulties in your relationships. It is important to talk about these feelings as it may help you see things more clearly and help you feel more in control of your situation.

As The British Heart Foundation notes in *Heart Valve Surgery*, following heart surgery, most hospitals invite patients and their partners/family to join a cardiac rehabilitation program. The program usually includes exercise sessions and advice on lifestyle including healthy eating and relaxation techniques, aiming to rebuild your confidence and restore you to as full a life as possible.

Going to *cardiac rehabilitation classes* (next chapter) gives you the opportunity to ask questions and talk about any worries you may have and to meet other patients and their families. If you find it difficult to attend a rehabilitation program, you may be offered a self-help "Heart Manual" (a home-based rehabilitation manual) from your local hospital to use at home.

You may also find it helpful to join a "heart support group", as it can be useful to talk with people who have been through similar experiences. Some groups hold exercise classes and invite speakers to talk on medical as well as general topics.

For example, during my recovery I learned of Mended Hearts. Mended Hearts is a national nonprofit organization affiliated with the American Heart Association. It has been offering support to heart surgery patients, their families and caregivers for more than 50 years. Recognized for its role in facilitating a positive patient-care experience, Mended Hearts partners with 460 hospitals and rehabilitation clinics and offers services to heart patients through visiting programs, support group meetings and educational forums.

Because Mended Hearts is made up of the very kinds of people it serves—heart patients, their families, and others impacted by heart disease – its members draw on personal experience as they help others. Mended Hearts Support Groups help people understand that there can be a rich, rewarding life after heart challenges. Members can listen, share their experiences, learn from healthcare professionals and volunteer to talk to other heart patients about what they may face including lifestyle changes, depression, recovery, and treatment. Annually, Mended Hearts volunteers make 227,000 hospital visits to patients and 30,000 visits to family members and caregivers.

Former Valve Surgery Patient Quote: Kathy Benson (Minnesota)

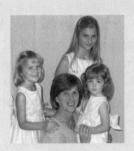

"Don't gauge your surgery and recovery on others. Each surgery is unique and each person will handle things in a different manner. It seems patients strive to become *normal* as fast as they can. What is *normal*? We will forever be heart surgery patients."

17

The Recovery Gets Back On Track

In this chapter, you will:
- Learn some additional steps to help your recovery stay on track.
- Understand the physical and mental benefits of going to a cardiac rehabilitation program.
- Review survey results specific to cardiac rehabilitation and professional counseling.

Following my realization that I needed help for cardiac depression, I took several steps to get my recovery back on track – both physically and mentally. I was now in my seventh week following surgery and I needed professional help to further my recovery.

Here are the steps I took:

1. **I returned to my cardiologist and my surgeon to make sure everything was physically okay with me.**

2. **I saw a pain management specialist, Dr. Robert Swift, in Manhattan Beach, California.**

3. **I entered a twelve-week cardiac rehabilitation program at Torrance Memorial Hospital in Los Angeles.**

4. **I entered individual therapy with a psychologist trained in cardiac rehabilitation.**

Together, these four steps worked wonders on my brain and body.

I now had people, processes and technology guiding my recovery.

I was no longer alone with my thoughts and feelings. I was no longer alone with my physical rehabilitation. It felt great to no longer be alone with detrimental self-thought.

My recovery was getting back on course.

"There's Nothing Wrong With Me!"

Momentum was building. Slowly, I started to develop an answer to the question that had been nagging me for weeks.

As you may remember (from Chapter 16) that question was, *"What's wrong with me?"*

The more I talked with doctors, the more I talked with nurses, the more I talked with fellow patients, the answer to that question appeared.

Nothing.

Nothing was wrong with me!

However, there was no way I could comprehend that reality because I did not have the *right* information and the *right* interactions to generate that thought.

A big mental light-bulb had gone off!

My Saving Grace... Cardiac Rehabilitation

While all of the steps listed above were helpful in getting me out of depression, I believe that entering a cardiac rehab program was the most critical step to enhancing my recovery.

I entered the Cardiac Rehabilitation Program at Torrance Memorial on February

24, 2006. I had no expectations. All I knew was that my chest was tight, tense and in pain.

I was stiff as a board. I really needed help restoring my physical confidence.

I entered the cardiac rehab facility to find it operating at full-speed.

Bike pedals were spinning. Treadmills were spinning. Rowing machines were spinning.

There, in front of me, was action.

In total, fifteen patients were moving, talking and laughing. Heart monitors rested on the chests of each patient.

Some patients were sweating.

Some patients were stretching.

Some patients were lifting weights.

My gut immediately told me I had found something special.

Several nurses – Donna, Debbie, Sherri, Socorro, Sidney aand Karey – were running the show. That day, Debbie manned the controls at the front-desk, which acted like the central nervous system of the facility. From her desk, Debbie could remotely monitor the heart rhythms of each patient wearing a heart monitor.

At random intervals, Debbie would call out "Crank it up!" to a patient. I would learn that call phrase was one of many indicators for a patient to take a specific action. "Crank it up!" indicated that a patient's warm up was complete and that he or she should now increase their activity to increase their heart rate. One of the more funny indicators was "Strip and stretch!"

It was a stimulating environment.

As I walked in, Debbie looked at me, smiled and said, "You must be Adam!"

Considering that I was twenty years younger than most of her patients, Debbie had an easy time separating me from the other patients starting that day.

Over the next hour, I was reintroduced to physical exercise. Within the first few minutes, I was peddling away on a stationary bike. Then, I was put on a treadmill. I ended the session with a ten-minute stretch.

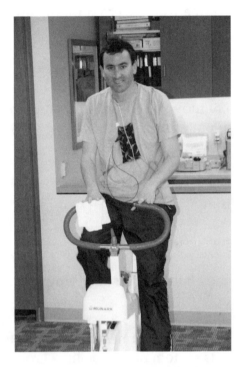

At Torrance Memorial's Cardiac Rehab Program
(Source: Doug Pick)

In addition to the physical element of cardiac rehab, I immediately began to realize another important part of the program – interacting with my fellow patients.

For the first time, I was spending time with other heart valve surgery patients - talking about my situation and talking about their situation, talking about my problems and talking about their problems.

I was relating in a new way with a new group of people.

With each cardiac rehab session, my mind eased and body strengthened.

Talking With Ted And Don, Heart Valve Surgery Patients

Ted was one of the first cardiac rehab patients I met to *really* make me feel better.

Ted had a heart valve repair about four weeks before my operation. Ted needed an urgent valve repair at the age of forty-two years. It completely caught him off-guard.

I told him my story - about the pain, the Vicodin and the depression. He laughed and said, "Yep. I know exactly how you feel. I was the same way."

Don, a retired physics teacher, had a mechanical heart valve replacement. We had surgery during the same week in December, 2005. So, we really compared notes.

Don said to me one day, "Does your chest ever crack or click?"

I was ecstatic to hear that question. I previously thought my chest cracking was a sign that my sternum was unstable.

"Yes!" I exclaimed in relief.

He smiled and said, "Me too!"

Then Don threw me a curve ball, "But ya know what... It cracked before my operation."

Don was right. My chest cracked before the operation as well.

I was in heaven at cardiac rehab.

Don't get me wrong, it was uncomfortable at times. But, I could feel my chest getting stronger and my confidence returning.

What Do The Experts Say About Cardiac Rehab?

Commenting on the impact of cardiac rehab, Dr. Robert J. Matthews, a cardiologist and internal medicine physician in Los Angeles, notes:

> Although cardiac rehabilitation programs are usually thought of as primarily exercise programs, they also offer psychological benefits that tend to help resolve transient depression. With many special medical conditions, other patients who have been through the experience can provide meaningful psychological support.

There is empathy among the members and they encourage each other. Patients who have participated in a comprehensive rehabilitation program are more likely to return to work and to report a more satisfactory quality of life. Patients who are deemed ineligible for an exercise program may be the ones needing more psychological counseling.

Survey Results – Cardiac Rehabilitation And Therapy

Given my positive experience in cardiac rehabilitation and the research provided above, I was surprised to learn that 49% of patients surveyed did not take advantage of the benefits provided by cardiac rehab programs. As shown in our survey, only 51% of heart valve surgery patients joined cardiac rehab programs.

Did You Join A Cardiac Rehabilitation Program Following Heart Valve Surgery?
(Source: www.Heart-Valve-Surgery.com)

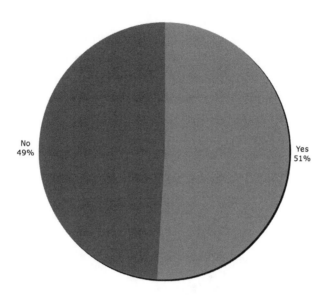

No
49%

Yes
51%

Personally, I believe this is a huge issue with heart valve surgery recovery. In my opinion, the benefits of cardiac rehabilitation programs are invaluable to the patient. That said, I strongly encourage you or your loved one to research rehabilitation programs in your area before, during or immediately following surgery.

As you read earlier in this chapter, I also entered a professional counseling program to help get my recovery back on track. For eight weeks, I individually met with a psychologist who specialized in cardiac surgery recovery.

Those hour-long sessions were very powerful.

There were tears and there were smiles in those sessions.

Some days I wept like a baby.

Other days I was immune to Kleenex. On those days, I trumpeted my successes (walking, stretching, driving, lifting weights, swimming, making dinner, getting off Vicodin and having sex again).

In fact, it was in one of those sessions that the idea for this book came about.

Again, I was surprised to learn that individual therapy was not prevalent among former, heart valve surgery patients surveyed. Only six of sixty-five patients (9%) participated in professional counseling following surgery.

**Did You Require Any Form Of Counseling Or Therapy Following Surgery?
(Source: www.Heart-Valve-Surgery.com)**

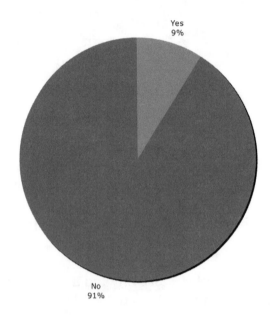

Yes
9%

No
91%

After 57 Cardiac Rehab Sessions, Charles Feels "Very Fortunate"

Adam's Heart Valve Surgery Blog Excerpt – Posted May 31, 2009

When talking with patients and caregivers about heart surgery recovery, I can never say enough about cardiac rehabilitation programs. I hear from patients over-and-over-and-over-and-over again about how valuable cardiac rehabilitation programs are for their physical, social and mental well-being after heart surgery.

Here's a quick note I just received from Charles Harrall, an active 65-year old businessman from Nevada, about cardiac rehab, goal setting and medication management. Charles writes:

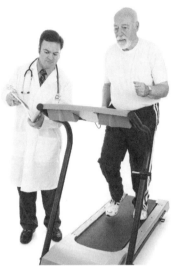

Hi Adam,

I am one year past my aortic valve replacement, mitral valve repair and triple bypass.

I took your advice to heart (pun intended) and I went to cardiac rehab... 57 times!!! I think I am doing great now because I had my goals and achieved them.

When I came home from the hospital I was taking 9 medications. Plus, I was on oxygen. Now, I am down to 3 medications with dosages that are 50% less than they were. I am 65 and very fortunate that I had a great doctors and excellent care. I also realized doctors can only help people who are willing to help themselves.

Your heart valve surgery book helped me take charge of my health and have successful results.

God Bless!

Charles Harrall

chapter

18

One Year After Heart Valve Surgery

As I write these words, it is one year after my aortic and pulmonary valve replacements.   It's amazing how much can change in twelve months.

Regarding the heart valve surgery, I do my best to use it as an inspirational tool. I have been given a *second chance* at life and I intend to make the most of it.

With that in mind, I proposed to Robyn on May 20, 2006. She said yes. We are now planning our wedding on July 7, 2007.   I could not have found a better person to partner-up with for this fun game called life.

In September of this year, I went to Europe for two weeks on business. I was in seven countries in thirteen days. It was a personal triumph for me. Being away that long, only nine months after open-heart surgery, illustrates that anything is possible.

So you know, I returned to work three and a half months after heart valve surgery. I strongly encourage you to <u>not</u> rush back to the office. If possible, take the time you need to adjust. And, when you do return to work, ask your manager (boss) if you can go half-time for the first week.

 Although I did not mention it earlier, I lost 15 pounds following my operation. I gained it all back and then some. In fact, I think I'm going to start a diet tomorrow.

As for my heart? Good news! Good news!

I recently saw my cardiologist (Ben Rosin, Torrance Memorial) for the one-year check-up. The echocardiogram came back very positive. Dr. Rosin said, "I'm very delighted with this. I don't need to see you for two years. Now, get out of here and go have some fun!"

I'm taking that advice to *heart*.

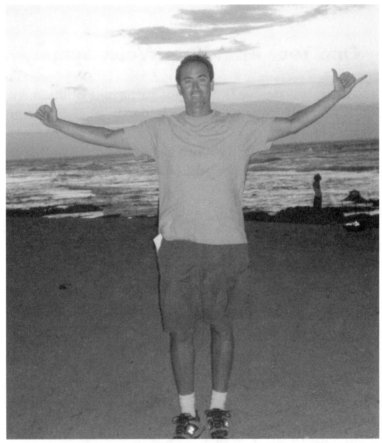

Adam Pick In Hawaii, Ten Months After Surgery
(Source: Robyn Pick)

Survey Results – Looking Back On Heart Valve Surgery

As you have read in this book, my heart valve surgery experience was riddled with ups and downs. Some might say that heart valve surgery can be similar to a rollercoaster.

Still, I am convinced that this experience has gifted me new perspective on life, love, family and friends. So you know, I often refer to my post-operative life as a *second chance*. Even with the pain, the Vicodin addiction and the cardiac depression, I know this surgery has been a positive influence in my life.

That said, I was curious to know what other patients felt about their heart valve surgery experience in retrospect. So, I asked fifty patients about their feelings towards heart valve surgery.

Specifically, I asked the former patients, "On a scale of 1 (negative change) to 10 (positive change), how would you score the impact of heart valve surgery on your life?"

The results of the survey were quite amazing. Over 45% of patients surveyed, responded with the highest possible score of 10... A positive change!

I guess I'm not the only one who looks back on their heart valve surgery experience positively.

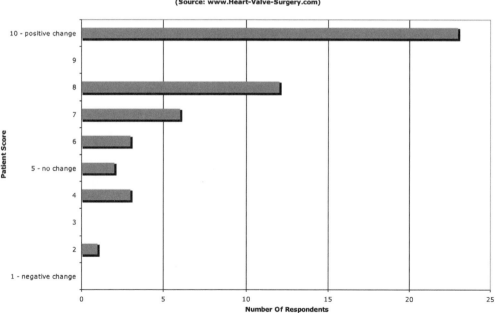

19

The Best Piece Of Advice

Ever since my operation, I have interacted with many patients preparing for heart valve surgery. One of the most frequent questions I receive is, "What is the best piece of advice you can share with me prior to heart valve surgery?"

In answering that question, I found myself stumped time and time again. I could not think of just one answer to that question. Perhaps that is why I wrote this book – to share many pieces of advice to those preparing for heart valve surgery.

Considering my lack of a 'best piece of advice', I decided to ask fifty, former heart valve surgery patients that exact same question during a recent survey. I was very curious to see how they would respond to the question I could not answer.

Here, for your review, is a select set of survey responses to the question, "What is the best piece of advice you can share with me prior to heart valve surgery?"

"Take all the time off of work that you can. I was back at my desk three weeks post-operation. I went full-time after four weeks. BIG MISTAKE!"
- James Widmer (Oregon)

"Always get another opinion. Don't be afraid to ask lots of questions. Always try to keep a positive attitude on getting better... and prayer does work."
- Sandra Shields (Kansas)

"Don't gauge your surgery and recovery on others. Each surgery is unique and each person will handle things in a different manner. It seems patients strive to become *normal* as fast as they can. What is *normal*? We will forever be heart surgery patients."

- Kathy Benson (Minnesota)

"I found it extremely helpful to practice relaxation techniques (deep breathing exercises, muscle relaxation, etc) in the weeks prior to surgery. It only took about 20 minutes a day and I think it allowed me to be much more calm on the day of the surgery and during my recovery. I experienced none of the irrational anger or frustration that many heart patients describe during recovery."

- Kate Leeman (Ohio)

"Don't get discouraged the first few days after surgery. It is normal to feel very weak and to feel nauseous at the beginning. Just let people help you at the beginning and you will see the progress each day."

- Adrienne de Burgos (Quebec)

"Ask questions."

- Jackie Pancoat (California)

"Don't be frightened. If you die during the surgery you are not going to know anything about it and if you don't have the surgery you are going to die anyway; so, there is no point worrying about it. Get your affairs in order then relax. Stressing and worrying about having the surgery isn't going to help you or your loved ones."

- Sue Monks (United Kingdom)

"Don't be afraid to ask questions. No question is un-important as long as it helps you to get ready for things to come. Read as much as you can to become as familiar with circumstances and procedures and options. The better prepared you are... The better your experience will be."

- DeWayne Epley (Georgia)

"Get as much information as you can before making any decisions."

- LeRoy Schmidt (Ontario, Canada)

"Question everything until you get the answers that you need."

- Marla Brenner (Pennsylvania)

"Don't give up! Patience, Patience, Patience."

- Hayley Irwin (Nevada)

"Read up on the procedure, do your homework, ask questions during your visits with both the surgeon and other doctors. Don't be afraid to ask for most anything while in the hospital. Treat the nurses with respect and it will be repaid in kind. SPEAK UP when you feel something isn't right or is uncomfortable. Humans make mistakes. Manage pain, do not let it manage you. OOOOPS!!! That's more than one piece of advice!!!"

- Danny Mitchell (Georgia)

"It isn't as bad as your imagination makes it."

- Karen (Florida)

"Research as much as possible prior to the surgery.... Even watch live surgeries on the Internet. I found in doing all that research... There were absolutely no surprises."

- Jack Schommer (Ohio)

"Try to look at how great the quality of life will be after surgery. Focus on the positive."

- Cheryl Bambery (Massachusetts)

Former Valve Surgery Patient Quote:
Taylor Browning (California)

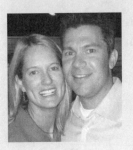

"Today, I turned 36 years old and my ascending aorta and aortic valve turned a very young 22 days old! I told someone earlier that I can take the average... So, I guess I'm about 18. I feel great!"

Heart Valve Surgery Survey Results

As you have already seen in *The Patient's Guide To Heart Valve Surgery*, an extensive survey was conducted with more than sixty-five, former heart valve surgery patients and caregivers.

This survey was performed to better understand the realities and impact of heart valve surgery upon patients and their respective caregivers.

While the survey is on-going, the initial results of that survey already appear to illustrate several opinions, trends and feelings about heart valve surgery from the patient and caregiver perspective.

Here is a quick summary of the survey results already presented in *The Patient's Guide To Heart Valve Surgery*:

- Only 35% of patients acquired a second opinion to confirm their valve defect or disease prior to surgery.

- Valve surgery is known to impact all age groups. However, our study illustrated that the 31-45 and the 46-60 age groups were most prevalent among respondents.

- On a scale of 1 (negative) to 10 (excellent), 62% of surgeons received the highest possible score of 10 for their bedside manner.

- The average time in the hospital for heart valve surgery patients was *five days*.

- Eighty percent of patients felt their hospital experience could be categorized as *good* or *excellent*.

- The majority of patients felt heart valve surgery recovery was *more difficult than expected.*

- The average time which patients returned to work following surgery was 4 to 10 weeks; however, many patients did not return to work until 15 weeks post-operation.

- Fifty one percent (51%) of patients joined cardiac rehabilitation programs.

- Only nine percent (9%) of patients entered individual therapy or professional counseling following heart valve surgery.

- On a scale of 1 (negative change) to 10 (positive change), the majority of respondents felt heart valve surgery had a positive impact on their lives.

In addition to the results already provided in *The Patient's Guide To Heart Valve Surgery*, here are several, other survey results from our study.

True or False: My Surgeon And Cardiologist Fully Prepared Me For Heart Valve Surgery Recovery.
(Source: www.Heart-Valve-Surgery.com)

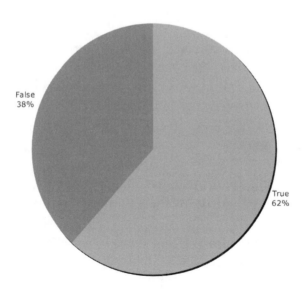

False
38%

True
62%

Did You Travel Outside Your Hometown (More Than 2 Hours) To Arrive At The Hospital?
(Source: www.Heart-Valve-Surgery.com)

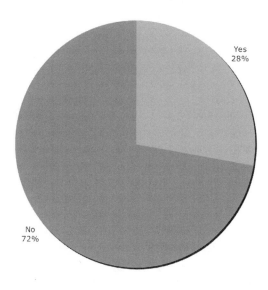

Yes
28%

No
72%

Are You On Medication Following Heart Valve Surgery?
(Source: www.Heart-Valve-Surgery.com)

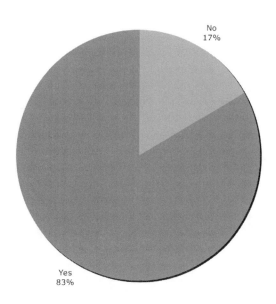

No
17%

Yes
83%

Question: What types of medication are you using following heart valve surgery?

- Coreg, Lipitor, Plavix, Aspirin, Altace
- Aspirin
- Atenolol, Aspirin
- Coumadin (Jantovin), Lasix, Digoxin, Spernolactone, Coreg, Atacand
- Atenalol, Warfarin
- Coumadin
- Atenolol 25 mg
- Coumadin and Coreg
- Warfarin, Toprol XL, Spironolactone, Lisinopril
- Cordarone and Coreg plus the usual litany of blood pressure medicines including Lasix
- Toprol and Lisinopril
- Warfarin, Amiodorone
- Amiodarone, Lopressor
- Norvasc, HCTZ, Aspirin
- Coumadin, Lopressor, DiazideHCT, Lipitor
- A long list (10) including Prozac
- Warfarin, Toprol XL, Crestor

Do You Feel Your Stay In The Hospital Was Long Enough?
(Source: www.Heart-Valve-Surgery.com)

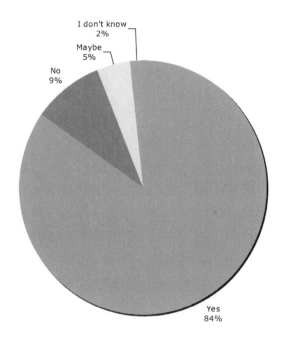

I don't know
2%

Maybe
5%

No
9%

Yes
84%

On A Scale Of 1 (Problematic) To 10 (Excellent) How Would You Score Your Surgeon's Willingness
To Communicate Information About Your Procedure And Listen To Your Concerns?
(Source: www.Heart-Valve-Surgery.com)

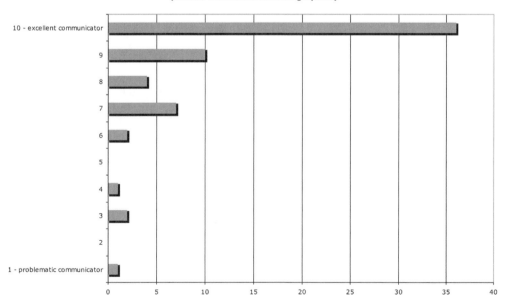

Question: Did you experience any perceived form of complication following heart valve surgery?

Answer: Many patients responded that they experienced some form of complication after their surgical experience. Perceived complications addressed by patients include:

- Anxiety
- Atrial fibrillation
- Blurred vision
- Collarbone pain
- Deep breathing pain
- Depression
- Dizziness
- Dressler's Syndrome
- Erectile dysfunction
- Fatigue
- Fluid in lungs
- Headaches
- Heart palpitations
- High heart rates
- Hoarse voice
- Insomnia
- Memory loss
- Nerve damage
- Night Sweats
- Pain
- Pneumonia
- Pounding heart sensations
- Problems sleeping at night
- Stroke
- Ventricular tachycardia
- Vertigo

chapter 21

Open Heart Surgery Recovery Update – Surf's Up!

Blog Posting From www.Heart-Valve-Surgery.com - Tuesday, March 6th, 2007
By Adam Pick

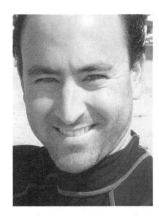

On December 21, 2005, nearly 435 days ago, I had open-heart surgery to fix a congenital defect in the aortic valve of my heart.

After thirty-four years of life, my bicuspid aortic valve, which suffered from stenosis and regurgitation, needed to be replaced.

As many of you know, this open-heart medical operation (known as the Ross Procedure) triggered a series of challenging lows (e.g. cardiac depression) and a series of memorable highs (e.g. my engagement to Robyn).

Well… Two days ago, I experienced another memorable high that I wanted to share with you - my friends, family, readers and blog subscribers.

"What happened?!" you may be wondering as you see my smiling, much in need of a shave, face.

This past Saturday, I dug my dusty, nine-foot, eight-inch McTavish surfboard out of the garage. Then, I reached into the dark corner of my closet and grabbed my RipCurl wetsuit.

Yep…

It was time to complete my physical recovery from heart valve surgery.

It was time to surf again.

The day was a surfers dream. Sunny, with a few swooshes of cloud in the blue skies above. I think the temperature in Los Angeles on Saturday was around 80 degrees Fahrenheit.

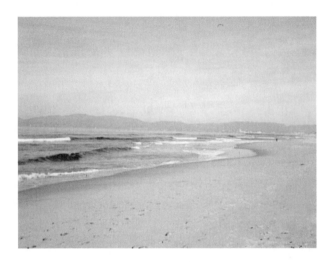

The Pacific Ocean held to its name. It was symbolically calm and glassy.

And the waves…

The waves were as playful as a six-week old puppy.

Perfect for a longboarder like me…

Or, more accurately, perfect the longboarder I remembered to be prior to my surgery.

With booties strapped on, I entered the cold, salt water with no expectations.

This would be my first time on a surfboard in eighteen months. This would be the first time that my new heart would experience a surfing adrenaline shot. This would be the first time that my stitched sternum would feel forces

controlled by the one-and-only Mother Nature.

Come to think of it, I was a surfing virgin again.

Fear and anxiety bubbled up as my chest smacked down on the white, waxed fiberglass board. I started to paddle.

"As long as I don't break," I thought to myself, "Everything will be fine."

Fifteen feet into my initial paddle, however, that thought transformed.

There was no pain in my chest. There was no discomfort in my nine-inch scar. There were no heart palpitations that I could feel. There was nothing but a boundary-less emotion of joy.

Chilly water splashed overhead as I slipped through an oncoming wave. More chilly water from the next wave and the next. About a minute after entering the water, I was outside the breaking waves amongst the other surfers in the line-up.

"Is this really happening?" I thought to myself. "This must be some kind of wonderful dream."

I tested my chest once again.

Using my hands, I thrust my body upward to strike the traditional, surfer pose you see as you drive along Pacific Coast Highway in Malibu – butt on the board, legs on the side, chest slumped but upright, eyes gazing to the water's horizon.

Again, no pain...

Hmmmmmmmm.....

"Don't get cocky Adam," I thought to myself, "Take it easy... You did not come out here to go nuts. Just get used to your surfboard. Paddle around a little. Then, call it a day. You've been through a lot."

Needless to say, that thought disappeared.

In its place, came an empowering voice that screamed aloud, "LET'S HAVE SOME FUN!!!"

In the distance, I saw a friendly mound of bulging water that was going to peak about twenty feet to my right.

Instinct took over.

The time was now.

The hunt was on.

Nanoseconds later I was paddling to the peak.

"GO! GO! GO! GO! CHARGE! CHARGE! CHARGE!" the empowering voice was now yelling in my head. Like a windmill, my arms circulated, cutting through the water, powering me forward.

And then...

It happened....

The water's powerful energy transferred to my surfboard.

The need to paddle disappeared.

I angled to the right.

There was only one thing left to do...

One thing.

My internal cheerleader rose again and rang-out, "UP!"

I lept to my feet.

I was surfing again.

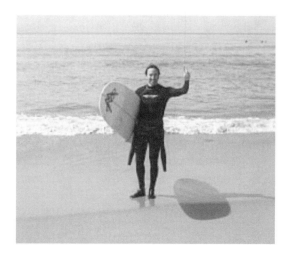

I would spend the next 45 minutes frolicking in the water with my friend Jeff. (Jeff recently had a heart attack and had three stents inserted. Already, two months into Jeff's recovery, he's surfing. How incredible is that?!)

The magic of the day extended when thirty dolphins showed up to celebrate with us.

We had our own surf party to celebrate my recovery and my belated 35th birthday.

Thanks to each of you for your support and encouragement. I'm not sure where I would be if not for your love and help during my recovery!!!

Keep on tickin!

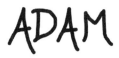

REFERENCES:

The Cleveland Clinic (http://www.clevelandclinic.org)

Edwards Lifesciences, Andrew Karplus, Clay Donne (http://www.edwards.com)

The Texas Heart Institute (http://www.texasheartinstitute.org)

National Heart Lung And Blood Institute (http://www.nhlbi.nih.gov)

Servier International (http://www.servier.com)

The Mayo Clinic (http://www.mayoclinic.com)

Medtronic (http://www.medtronic.com)

Cedar-Sinai Medical Center (www.csmc.edu)

Healthgrades (http://www.healthgrades.com)

U.S. News And World Report (http://www.usnews.com)

Cardiothoracic Surgery Network (http://www.ctsnet.org)

Keck School Of Medicine (http://www.usc.edu)

Columbia University (http://www.columbia.edu)

National Library Of Medicine (http://www.nlm.nih.gov)

East Carolina University (http://www.ecu.edu)

Blue Shield Insurance Company (http://www.blueshieldca.com)

Purdue Pharma (http://www.purduepharma.com)

Merz Pharma (http://www.merz.com)

Mitchell, Dr. R. Scott (http://www.stanford.edu)

Fogoros, Dr. Richard, Why Cardiac Depression Is So Common? (http://heartdisease.about.com/mbiopage.htm)